# VITAMINS DEFICIENCY SYMPTOMS & CURES

## MODERN DEFICIENCY ILLNESSES

Using the SpectraCell Intracellular Micronutrient Panel

BY

DAN PURSER MD AND JARED LARKIN

# FOREWORD

Vitamin deficiency symptoms have been a frequent topic of discussion around our dinner table as the kids in our house grow up. For this reason, Jared Larkin and I chose to cover this topic as other families may have similar questions, but do not have resources to find solutions.

Jared is currently a pre-med student at Brigham Young University who started the idea of this book. He performed all the research of the benefits of the vitamins and studies while also supplying majority of the references. During our time together writing this book, we had many discussions on how technology has influenced our thoughts on vitamins and medicine in general. One of the forms of technology we will cover in this book is a SpectraCell® blood test.

Jared's love for medicine comes from his family history beginning with his maternal grandfather. He originally came from Tampico, Mexico and was sponsored across the border as a university student at the UCLA School of Medicine. Later, he did two tours of duty on US Naval ships during the Korean War as a ship's doctor. After the war, he didn't practice medicine, but started work in the growing Southern California biotech industry of building and designing hyperbaric oxygen beds. He ended up in the last half of his life teaching in the university system in Southern California while living in Santa Ana, California with his wife.

Jared and I hope you enjoy this book as much as we have enjoyed writing it. Solutions for vitamin deficiencies exist and we want this book to be a great resource of knowledge for you and your family.

—Dan Purser MD

# TABLE OF CONTENTS

# INTRODUCTION

Living in modern America, vitamin deficiencies aren't the first problems we think of with our health. However, recent trends indicate these deficiencies are becoming a larger issue, especially for those who have been on a hardcore, long-term diet. Surprisingly, I see cases caused from vitamin deficiencies such as scurvy, pernicious anemia, pseudo-hypothyroidism, pseudo-diabetes, color blindness, night blindness, depression, and fatigue. When I was fresh out of medical school and residency 30 years ago, I would not have believed treating these deficiencies would resolve these conditions. I continue to be a licensed, practicing physician while exploring natural solutions to determine the best treatments for my patients' conditions. Fortunately, I continue to see results in my patients who have suffered for years by treating these root causes easily overlooked by other physicians. As I see more of my patients continually improve from these natural approaches, my belief in naturopathic medicine grows stronger every day.

Throughout this book, Jared and I reference SpectraCell® several times. Please note that we are not affiliated with SpectraCell® nor receive monetary compensation for this book. I was fortunate to learn of SpectraCell® years ago as it is an FDA- and HHS-approved intracellular technology. SpectraCell® has helped me determine vitamin levels in patients' white blood cells accurately and efficiently countless times.

If the information found in this book can help at least one person, Jared and I find the many hours dedicated writing this book worthwhile. If you have other questions or would like to schedule an appointment, feel free to contact our office at (801) 796-7667 or info@danpursermd.com.

God bless and go in good health,
Dan Purser MD & Jared Larkin

# CHAPTER ONE:
## How Vitamins Can Be Obtained Naturally

Many patients ask me how vitamins can be increased naturally to overcome deficiencies. Although this process can be long and hard, I recommend taking the supplement route for the first three to six months. For example, patients with severe homozygous forms of MTHFR cannot get enough methylcoblamin or methylfolate in their diet. Therefore, in order to make up for their deficiencies, baseline support supplements are used. Below are ways to incorporate essential vitamins for these deficiencies:

## B COMPLEX VITAMINS

- B1 Thiamin
    - Nutritional Yeasts, Rice Bran, Wheat Germ, Pork, Legumes (beans, peas, soybeans, lentils), Enriched Grain & Grain Products (cereals)

- B2 Riboflavin
    - Nutritional Yeasts, Meats, Dairy Products, Green Leafy Vegetables, Grain Products & Enriched Grains

- B3 Niacinamide
    - Nutritional Yeasts, Meats, Legumes (including peanuts), Enriched Cereals & Potatoes

- B6 Pyridoxine
    - Nutritional Yeasts, Potatoes, Meats, Wheat Germ, Bananas, Legumes, Fortified Cereal Products

- B12 Cobalamin
  - Dietary sources for cobalamins are strictly from animal foodstuffs as Vitamin B12 is not found in plant foodstuffs.

- Folate
  - Legumes, Vitamin-Fortified Cereals, Green Leafy Vegetables, Wheat Germ, Seeds, Nuts & Liver

- Pantothenate
  - Nutritional Yeasts, Meats, Legumes, Whole Grain Products, Wheat Germ, Vegetables, Nuts & Seeds

- Biotin (See Vitamin B8)
  - Liver, Egg Yolks, Nutritional Yeast, Royal Jelly, Legumes, Rice Bran, Whole Grains & Fish

## AMINO ACIDS

- Serine
  - Found in high-protein foods

- Glutamine
  - Found in high-protein foods, richest sources in milk, protein & meats

- Asparagine
  - Present in all proteins

## METABOLITES

- Choline
  - Lecithin, Choline Supplements, Egg Yolks, Liver, Soy Products, Wheat Germ, Peanuts and Legumes, Brain and Organ Meats, Potatoes & Lettuce

- Inositol
  - Whole Grains, Nuts, Seeds, Citrus Fruits, Cantaloupes & Organ Meats
- Carnitine
  - Red Meats, Pork, Seafood, Chicken & Dairy

## FATTY ACIDS

- Oleic Acid
  - Canola Oil, Olive Oil, Avocado Oil, Almond Oil, Avocados & High Oleic Safflower Oil

## OTHER VITAMINS

- D3 (Cholecalciferol)
  - Milk & Sunshine
- Vitamin A Retinol
  - Animal foods such as Whole Eggs, Milk, Liver, Fortified Breakfast Cereals, Cantaloupe, Apricots, Mango, Carrots, Spinach, Kale & Green Peas
- Vitamin K2
  - Kale, Beef Liver, Green Tea, Asparagus, Turnip Greens, Watercress, Spinach, Cheese, Broccoli, Oats, Lettuce, Peas, Cabbage & Whole Wheat

## MINERALS

- Calcium
  - Tofu, Milk and Dairy Products (milk, yogurt, cheeses), Bone Meal, Canned Salmon & Sardines (with bones)
- Manganese

- Whole Grains, Nuts, Leafy Vegetables, Pineapple & Teas
- Zinc
  - Oysters, Red Meats, Wheat Germ, Seeds, Nuts, Soybean Products, Legumes, Potatoes & Zinc-Fortified Cereal Products
- Copper
  - Oysters, Seeds, Avocados, Chick Peas, Dark Leafy Vegetables, Organ Meats, Dried Legumes, Whole Grain Breads, Nuts (almonds, hazelnuts, cashews in particular), Shellfish, Chocolate, Soybeans, Oats & Blackstrap Molasses
- Magnesium
  - Seeds (especially pumpkin), Nuts, Soybeans, Whole Grains, Potatoes, Legumes & Fresh Vegetables

## CARBOHYDRATE METABOLISM

- Glucose-insulin interaction
- Fructose Sensitivity
- Chromium
  - Whole Grains, Wheat Germ, Brewer's Yeast, Bran Cereal, Orange Juice, Romaine Lettuce, Raw Onions, Broccoli, Potatoes, Green Beans, Raw Tomatoes, Black Pepper, Grape Juice & Ham

## ANTIOXIDANTS

- Glutathione
  - Not absorbed well from foods, but can help with cysteine
- Cysteine

- Meats, Yogurt, Wheat Germ & Eggs
- CoQ10
  - Fish & Red Meat
- Selenium
  - Wheat Germ, Bran, Brazil Nuts, Red Swiss Chard, Whole Wheat Bread, Oats, Brown Rice & Turnips
- Vitamin E A-tocopherol
  - Almonds, Raw Seeds, Swiss Chard, Mustard Greens, Spinach, Turnip Greens, Kale, Plant Oils, Hazelnuts, Pine Nuts, Avocado, Broccoli, Parsley, Papaya & Olives
- Alpha Lipoic Acid
  - Organ Meats, Broccoli and Spinach, Brewer's Yeast, Brussels Sprouts, Peas & Tomatoes
- Vitamin C
  - Broccoli, Brussels Sprouts, Cantaloupe, Cauliflower, Citrus Fruits, Guava, Kiwi, Papaya, Parsley, Peas, Potatoes, Red and Green Peppers, Rose Hip, Strawberries & Tomatoes.

## IMMUNIDEX

"A patient's Immunidex™ score is one measurement to evaluate a person's cell-mediated immune system performance. Specifically, it measures T-cell lymphocyte proliferation. Since immune function is a systemic measure of general health, a higher Immunidex™ score is generally desired since it means a person can respond efficiently not only to exogenous threats such as pathogens or allergens, but also to endogenous threats like tumors. The immune system, comprised of both cell-mediated (Th1) and humoral (Th2) components, when balanced and performing optimally, affords us critical protection and promotes health and wellness.

Micronutrient deficiencies will undermine a person's immune function, and thus lower the Immunidex™. Since the highly complex immune system is dependent on the intracellular availability of vitamins, minerals and antioxidants, correcting specific micronutrient deficiencies typically raises the Immunidex™ and contributes to tangible clinical benefits, such as reduced infections and may assist in achieving Th1/Th2 balance."

- SpectraCell® website

SPECTROX

"The same technology also provides a total antioxidant function test (Spectrox™) which assesses the ability of cells to resist damage caused by free radicals and other forms of oxidative stress. Due to the considerable number of cellular antioxidants with extensive interactions, redundancies, repair and recharging capabilities, measuring total function is the most accurate and clinically useful way to assess your patients' capacity to resist oxidative damage."

- SpectraCell® website

## GLUCOSE-INSULIN INTERATION

"A stimulation of lymphocyte growth by insulin may indicate a functional deficiency of insulin in vivo, or a metabolic defect in glucose utilization. At suboptimal glucose concentrations, supplementation of lymphocyte cultures with insulin exerted a sparing effect. This means that insulin addition makes uptake or utilization of glucose and amino acids more efficient, producing more cellular energy, and thus, a greater growth response. At optimal concentrations of glucose, insulin does not exert a sparing effect in healthy persons."

- SpectraCell® website

## FRUCTOSE SENSITIVITY

"Humans have a limited ability to metabolize fructose (fruit sugar). Fructose is metabolized differently from other sugars. A fructose load leads to accumulation of fructose-1-phosphate in cells which may partially deplete intracellular ATP levels in susceptible individuals. Decreased cellular ATP causes disturbances in protein, DNA & RNA synthesis, interference with cyclic AMP formation, and reduced ammonia detoxification. Elevations of lactate, uric acid, and triglycerides may result with implications for gout and cardiovascular disease. Several forms of hereditary fructose intolerance have been described."

- SpectraCell® website

# CHAPTER TWO:
# A SPECTRACELL® RESULT

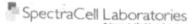SpectraCell Laboratories
Science • Health • Solutions

## LABORATORY REPORT

| Account Number: | Name: |
| --- | --- |
| Richard Steslow , D.O. | Gender: Male    DOB: 12/04/1990 |
| 2088 Ogden Ave. | |
| Ste 200 | Accession Number: |
| Aurora, IL 60504 | Requisition Number: |
| USA | |
| | Date of Collection:    10/05/2015 |
| | Date Received:    10/06/2015 |
| | Date Reported:    10/15/2015 |

### Summary of Deficient Test Results

Testing determined the following functional deficiencies:

| Vitamin B2 | Folate | Pantothenate | Serine |
| --- | --- | --- | --- |
| Glutamine | Glutathione | | |

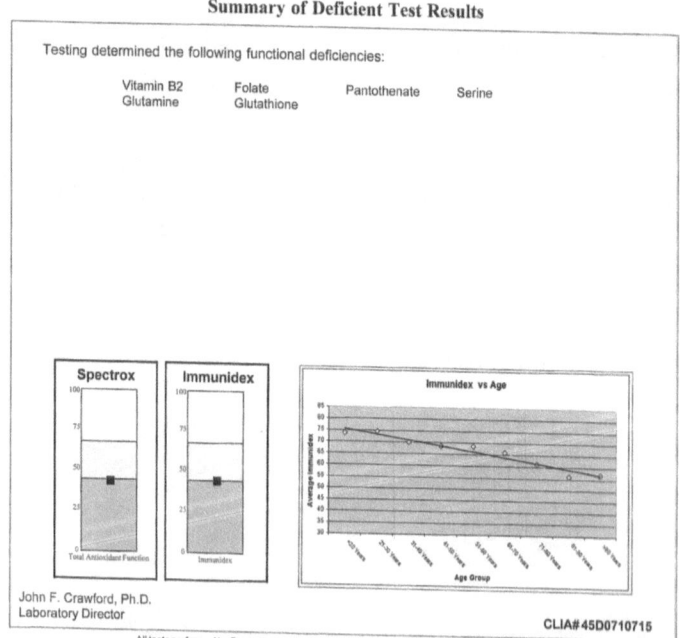

John F. Crawford, Ph.D.
Laboratory Director

CLIA# 45D0710715

All tests performed by SpectraCell Laboratories, Inc. • 10401 Town Park Drive Houston, TX 77072
Tel (713) 621-3101 • Toll-free (800)-227-LABS(5227) • Fax (713) 621-3234 • www.spectracell.com

SpectraCell Laboratories, Inc.
Laboratory Report

Accession Number:

## OVERVIEW OF TEST PROCEDURE

1. A mixture of lymphocytes is isolated from the blood.
2. These cells are grown in a defined culture medium containing optimal levels of all essential. nutrients necessary to sustain their growth in cell culture.
3. The T-lymphocytes are stimulated to grow with a mitogen (phytohemagglutinin) and growth is measured by the incorporation of tritiated (radioactive) thymidine into the DNA of the cells.

The growth response under optimal conditions is defined as 100%, and all other growth rates are compared to this 100% level of growth.

For example – we remove vitamin B6 from the medium and stimulate the cells to grow by mitogen stimulation. Growth is measured by DNA synthesis and the rate of growth is dependent only upon the functional level of vitamin B6 available within the cells to support growth. For Vitamin B6 a growth rate of at least 55% of the growth rate observed in the optimal (100%) media is considered normal. Results less than 55% are considered to indicate a functional deficiency for Vitamin B6. Each nutrient has a different reference range that was established by assaying thousands of apparently healthy individuals.

## BREAKING DOWN THE REPORT

### 1. TEST RESULT (% CONTROL)

This column represents the patient's growth response in the test media measured by DNA synthesis as compared to the optimal growth observed in the 100% media.

### 2. FUNCTIONAL ABNORMALS

An interpretation is provided for those nutrients found to be deficient.

### 3. REFERENCE RANGE

This column represents how this patient's result compares to thousands of patients previously tested. A patient's result is considered deficient when it is less than the reference range.

### 4. GRAPHS

The abnormal range of results is noted in the blue area. Abnormal results are indicated in red. The gray cross hatch area is a representation of the range of test results found in a random selection of subjects.

## SPECTROX® – TOTAL ANTIOXIDANT FUNCTION

SPECTROX® is a measurement of overall antioxidant function. The patient's cells are grown in the optimal media, stimulated to grow, and then increasing amounts of a free radical generating system (H2O2) are added. The cell's ability to resist oxidative damage is determined. The increasing levels of peroxide will result in diminished growth rates in those patients with poor antioxidant function capacity.

## INDIVIDUAL ANTIOXIDANT LEVELS

In the tests for individual antioxidants, it is determined which specific antioxidants may be deficient and thus affecting the SPECTROX® antioxidant function result. For these tests, the patient's cells are preincubated with one of the nutrient antioxidants, i.e. selenium, and then the Spectrox® test is repeated to determine if the addition of selenium improves the patient's antioxidant function. This process is repeated for each individual antioxidant.

Antioxidants tested with this process:
Glutathione, Cysteine, Coenzyme-Q10, Selenium, Vitamin E, Alpha Lipoic Acid, and Vitamin C.

SpectraCeil Laboratories, Inc.
Laboratory Test Report

Accession Number:

| Micronutrients | Patient Results (% Control) | Functional Abnormals | Reference Range (greater than) |
|---|---|---|---|
| **B Complex Vitamins** | | | |
| Vitamin B1 (Thiamin) | 88 | | >78% |
| Vitamin B2 (Riboflavin) | 51 | Deficient | >53% |
| Vitamin B3 (Niacinamide) | 88 | | >80% |
| Vitamin B6 (Pyridoxine) | 58 | | >54% |
| Vitamin B12 (Cobalamin) | 16 | | >14% |
| Folate | 28 | Deficient | >32% |
| Pantothenate | 6 | Deficient | >7% |
| Biotin | 54 | | >34% |
| | | | |
| **Amino Acids** | | | |
| Serine | 24 | Deficient | >30% |
| Glutamine | 36 | Deficient | >37% |
| Asparagine | 55 | | >39% |
| | | | |
| **Metabolites** | | | |
| Choline | 26 | | >20% |
| Inositol | 66 | | >58% |
| Carnitine | 54 | | >46% |
| | | | |
| **Fatty Acids** | | | |
| Oleic Acid | 72 | | >65% |
| | | | |
| **Other Vitamins** | | | |
| Vitamin D3 (Cholecalciferol) | 55 | | >50% |
| Vitamin A (Retinol) | 76 | | >70% |
| Vitamin K2 | 71 | | >30% |
| | | | |
| **Minerals** | | | |
| Calcium | 54 | | >38% |
| Manganese | 51 | | >50% |
| Zinc | 46 | | >37% |
| Copper | 53 | | >42% |
| Magnesium | 60 | | >37% |
| | | | |
| **Carbohydrate Metabolism** | | | |
| Glucose-Insulin Interaction | 56 | | >38% |
| Fructose Sensitivity | 36 | | >34% |
| Chromium | 55 | | >40% |
| | | | |
| **Antioxidants** | | | |
| Glutathione | 32 | Deficient | >42% |
| Cysteine | 55 | | >41% |
| Coenzyme Q-10 | 87 | | >86% |
| Selenium | 77 | | >74% |
| Vitamin E (A-tocopherol) | 89 | | >84% |
| Alpha Lipoic Acid | 88 | | >81% |
| Vitamin C | 63 | | >40% |
| | | | |
| **SPECTROX™** | | | |
| Total Antioxidant Function | 43 | | >40% |
| **Proliferation Index** | | | |
| Immunidex | 41 | | >40% |

*The reference ranges listed in the above table are valid for male and female patients 12 years of age or older.*

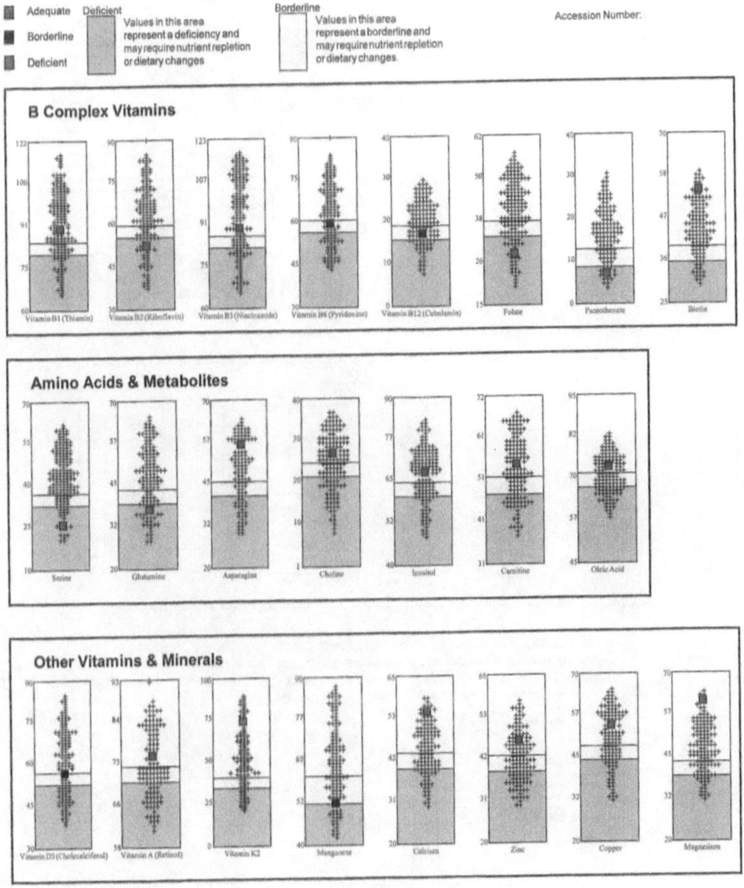

Adequate
Borderline
Deficient
Deficient
Values in this area represent a deficiency and may require nutrient repletion or dietary changes
Borderline
Values in this area represent a borderline and may require nutrient repletion or dietary changes.
Accession Number:
B Complex Vitamins
Vitamin B1 (Thiamin)
Vitamin B2 (Riboflavin)
Vitamin B3 (Niacinamide)
Vitamin B6 (Pyridoxine)
Vitamin B12 (Cobalamin)
Folate
Pantothenate
Biotin
Amino Acids & Metabolites
Serine
Glutamine
Asparagine
Choline
Inositol
Carnitine
Oleic Acid
Other Vitamins & Minerals
Vitamin D3 (Cholecalciferol)
Vitamin A (Retinol)
Vitamin K2
Manganese
Calcium
Zinc
Copper
Magnesium

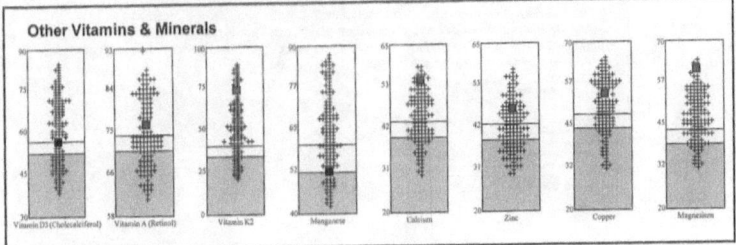

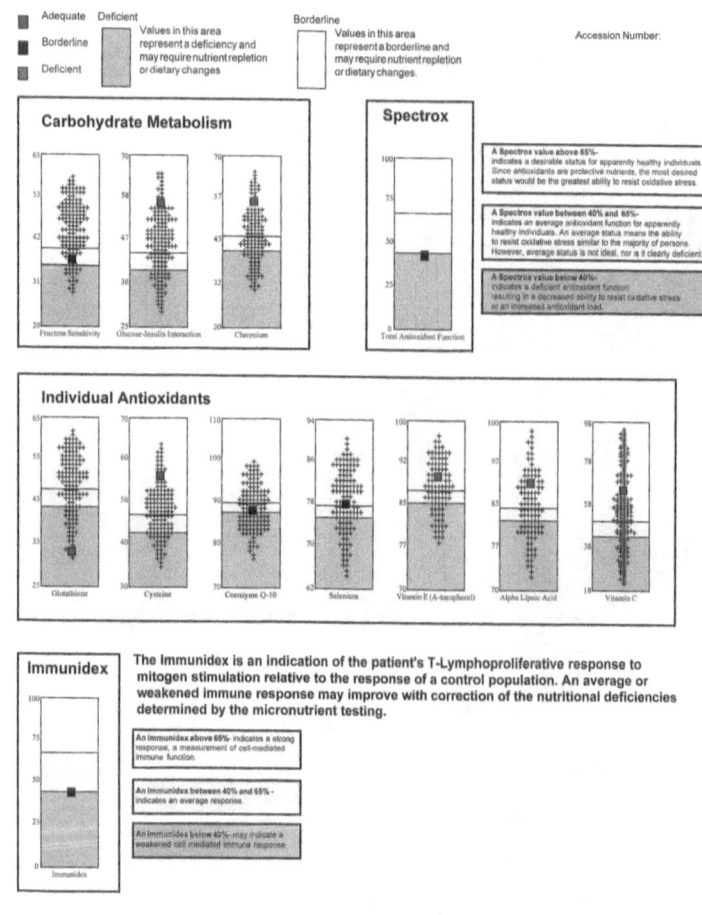

# CHAPTER THREE:
## TEN BENEFITS OF THIAMIN (B1)

- Helps with Dysmenorrhea.[1]

- Relieves the symptoms of PMS.[2]

- Helps with Herpetic itching.[3]

- Helps with glucose tolerance in those that have hyperglycemia.[4]

- Improves cardiac function in those that have chronic heart failure.[5]

- Reduces psychiatric stress and help those with sever alcohol abuse.[6]

- Helps stop the proliferation of cancer cells.[7] [8]

- Improves the cognitive functions of those with Alzheimer's.[9]

- Helps improve function in those that have Parkinson's.[10]

- Vitamin B1 deficiency leads to neurodegenerative diseases. Supplementation can help, if not stop, these diseases.[11]

## MY MEDICAL EXPERIENCE:

I have seen Type 2 diabetic patients (really had a thiamin deficiency) 'magically cured' after 90-100 days of therapy and patients in early congestive heart failure (CHF) suddenly get all better when I figured out it was a Vitamin B1 deficiency.

NOTE: This does not work for just anyone, you actually need to have a Vitamin B1 deficiency.

# CHAPTER FOUR:
## TEN BENEFITS OF RIBOFLAVIN (B2)

- Helps with migraine severity and frequency (when taken with magnesium and CoQ10).[12]

- Helps with burnout syndrome and improves energy.[13]

- Helps prevent radiotherapy related esophagitis.[14]

- Produces an antitumor effect.[15]

- Helps with the treatment of anemia and may be able to prevent it.[16]

- Helps with cardiovascular disease.[17]

- Strengthens the eyes and helps with keratoconus.[18]

- Kills bacteria topically as an antioxidant.[19]

- Improves the treatment of melanoma along with helping skin and hair health.[20]

- Improves wound healing and helps healing more rapidly.[21]

## MY MEDICAL EXPERIENCE:

I have seen many patients with intracellular Vitamin B2 (riboflavin) deficiencies and exhaustion/fatigue. However,

I have also seen exhaustion/fatigue caused both by a severe macrocytic anemia and a riboflavin deficiency (which also caused the anemia). After 100 days with treatment, my patients' anemia and exhaustion/fatigue were resolved.

NOTE: This does not work for just anyone, you actually must first have a B2 deficiency.

# CHAPTER FIVE:
## TEN BENEFITS OF NIACIN (B3)

- Lowers oxidative stress levels in those who have low HDL (high-density lipoprotein) levels, or lower cholesterol.[22]

- Improves lipid levels with extended release in those with Type 2 diabetes.[23]

- Improves erectile dysfunction in those with dyslipidemia.[24]

- Acts as a lipid-regulator on the bad lipids.[25]

- Helps with breast cancer and may reduce recurrence along with other supplements.[26]

- Aspirin and fruits containing pectin (apples) reduce the flushing induced by Niacin.[27]

- Helps lower triglycerides when HDL levels are low.[28]

- May decrease phosphorus, FGF23, and PTH concentrations in patients with chronic kidney disease.[29]

- Improves endothelial function and reverses plaque (with the proper statin) while preventing further vascular damage.[30]

- Niacin with laropiprant causes more adverse effects, without increasing cardiovascular health or strength.[31]

## MY MEDICAL EXPERIENCE:

In the first book I wrote on preventive medicine, we showed several niacin-plaque regression studies. In my practice, I have seen significant plaque regression and decreased cIMT (carotid intimal media thickness) occur in several patients who did not opt for the CABG bypass surgery. In addition to simvastatin, patients took 2,000mg of Vitamin B3 daily (required weeks to reach this dosage amount) along with significant flushing and following of liver function tests.

NOTE: A recent study shows plaque regression does not occur. However, I doubt the veracity of this one study compared to the fifty previous, well-done studies conducted.

# CHAPTER SIX:
## SIX BENEFITS OF CHOLINE (B4)

- Helps improve cognitive performance.[32]

- Choline intake is able to help prevent colorectal cancer.[33]

- Helps brain plasticity.[34]

- Helps with anxiety and depression.[35]

- Long-term supplementation of choline helps prevent cardiovascular disease.[36]

- For parents awaiting the birth of their children, findings indicate impaired choline metabolism showing a greater risk for DS, especially in a population associated with homocysteine-folate impairment.[37]

## MY MEDICAL EXPERIENCE:

The main time I see choline (B4) deficiencies is after patients with MTHFR get a SpectraCell® following treatment. Since most all these patients use our MTHFR base support product, most of their severe vitamin deficiencies are resolved as we try to correct the many pathway errors from MTHFR. I have not seen anything written about it, but I have also seen this deficiency occur with many other forms of MTHFR support products.

NOTE: Choline is synthesized by the human body, but not sufficiently to maintain good health. It is now considered an essential dietary nutrient and I find it to be a significant deficiency issue in people with MTHFR or MTRR.

# CHAPTER SEVEN:
## TEN BENEFITS OF PANTOTHENATE (B5)

- Improves cognition along with other micronutrients.[38]

- Improves periodontal wound healing with other B vitamins.[39]

- Increases wound healing post-tonsillectomy and lowers post-op related pain.[40]

- Alternative option to treat Atopic dermatitis Pantothenate along with hydrocortisone.[41]

- Pantothenate-based formulas act as a good skin moisturizer.[42]

- Dexpanthenol, a cosmetic form of Pantothenate, is a good substance that helps with skin disorders or injuries.[43]

- Lowers the risk of cardiovascular disease.[44]

- Lowers the frequency of epileptic seizures.[45]

- Helps in weight loss.[46]

˅   Pantothenic acid is an integral part of Coenzyme A

synthesis, without it can lead to neurodegenerative

diseases.[47]

## MY MEDICAL EXPERIENCE:

The most common problem I've seen with lack of pantothenate is poor wound healing. This is especially noticed with complex wound issues in a cosmetic surgery setting. I usually check intracellular vitamin levels with these cases via a SpectraCell® Micronutrient Panel to see these levels most accurately.

# CHAPTER EIGHT:
## TEN BENEFITS OF PYRIDOXINE (B6)

- Reduces nausea and vomiting for women during early pregnancy.[48]

- Controls premenstrual symptoms better along with calcium.[49]

- Overcomes infantile spasms and slows down relapses.[50]

- Stops and reverses some neurodegenerative diseases like Parkinson's Disease.[51]

- Exerts a carcinopreventive effect.[52]

- Helps and potentially alleviates symptoms for those with Carpal Tunnel Syndrome.[53]

- Acts as an antidepressant for those with depression along with other B vitamins.[54]

- Slows the atrophy of gray matter in the brain, Alzheimer's disease, and cognitive impairment along with other B vitamins.[55]

- Lowers the Total Plasma Homocysteine Concentrations in the blood along with other B vitamins.[56]

- Helps with Hand-foot syndrome during chemotherapy.[57]

## MY MEDICAL EXPERIENCE:

I have seen the occasional patients with nausea from either starting on our MTHFR base support product or from pregnancy. Both situations are quickly resolved when given a mild to moderate dose of pyridoxine (B6). Some deficiency cases treated with pyridoxine became much happier. They would tell me their long-standing depression had been resolved.

# CHAPTER NINE:
## TEN BENEFITS OF BIOTIN (B7)

- May have an impact on progressive MS.[58]

- Reduces Erythema, or skin rashes.[59]

- Relieves muscle cramps in patients undergoing hemodialysis.[60]

- Helps with Coronary risk factors along with chromium.[61]

- Helps with glycemic control.[62]

- Children with neurological issues, such as seizures, should be checked for biotin deficiency.[63]

- Helps with Uncombable Hair Syndrome.[64]

- Biotin deficiency leads to hair loss.[65]

- Helps with brittle nails.[66]

- Helps those with neurological disorders manage symptoms.[67]

## MY MEDICAL EXPERIENCE:

I have a number of women (and a few men) with severe hair loss learn they have a biotin deficiency (lack of zinc is a more common cause, but barely). After six months of therapy with biotin, their hair loss is almost always resolved, and they feel better.

# CHAPTER TEN:
## TEN BENEFITS OF INOSITOL (B8)

- Helps those who are bipolar with their depression and mania.[68]

- Lowers chance of diabetes in obese, pregnant women.[69]

- Increases sperm count in in men with infertility.[70]

- Relieves PCOS symptoms in women who have insulin resistance.[71]

- Helps with fertility in those who have PCOS or have tried ICSI.[72]

- Improves the success rates of IVF attempts.[73]

- Helps manage OCD.[74]

- Natural alternative to manage panic disorder.[75]

- Helps with Premenstrual Dysphoric Disorder.[76]

- Helps manage those who have bulimia or binge eating disorders.

## MY MEDICAL EXPERIENCE:

Inositol treatment results, when I treat a deficiency for this B vitamin, have been almost miraculous. Keep in mind there are several forms of this deficiency. One is D-Chiro-Inositol, or DCI, which can get rid of lifetime bipolar issues. The other is OCD behavior which is the more common myo-inositol. This therapy either works very quickly and clearly, or won't. When the therapy works, there is little doubt of the results and should be continued for a lifetime.

# CHAPTER ELEVEN:
## TEN BENEFITS OF FOLATE (B9)

NOTE: We are talking almost strictly about methyl folate, or folinic acid. Synthetic folic acid cannot be absorbed by most patients.

- Helps improve sperm viability and improves DNA integrity.[77]

- Supplementation of folate during child bearing years reduces the risk of neural tube defects, such as spina bifida, and helps in fetal development.[78]

- Reduces of stroke in adults with hypertension using folic acid.[79]

- Improves heart health and lowers cardiovascular risks along with other B vitamins.[80]

- Helps with prevention of colon cancer, while helping those who already have it.

- Reduces neuropathic pain for those with peripheral neuropathy along with B12.[81]

- Helps slow cognitive decline for those with mild cognitive impairment along with other B vitamins.[82]

- Deficiencies of folate and B vitamins lead to age-related macular degeneration.[83]

- Folate supplementation during pregnancy improves brain development of the child.[84]

- Helps manage long-term depression along with other B vitamins.[85]

## MY MEDICAL EXPERIENCE:

As with cobalamin (B12), I have seen more than a thousand intracellular folate deficiencies that experience a majority of these problems on the list above. A lack of folate is very common, especially those who have MTHFR. Unfortunately, if doctors can guess a folate deficiency for these patients, they often give them the synthetic folic acid which causes more problems. To compound the problem, the folic acid gives false, elevated serum levels because these patients cannot absorb it into their cells. Therefore, the folic acid piles up in their blood or serum.

# CHAPTER TWELVE:
## TEN BENEFITS OF COBALAMIN (B12)

- Improves cognitive impairment and poor memory for those who are B12 deficient.[86]

- Reduces the risk of stroke and dementia.[87]

- Reduces cardiovascular risk as those who are deficient in B12 usually have the TT MTHFR gene.[88]

- Improves strength and reduces symptoms of fatigue.[89]

- Those who are B12 deficient are more likely have depression.[90]

- Pernicious anemia is a cause of B12 deficiency and is treated by B12 shots or pills.[91]

- A B12 deficiency generally explains neuropsychiatric signs or symptoms.[92]

- Those with Type 2 diabetes are at an increased risk of B12 deficiency.[93]

- B12 deficiency is a cause of IBD and anemia.[94]

ﹾ Helps those with myalgic encephalomyelitis (ME) and

Fibromyalgia.[95]

## MY MEDICAL EXPERIENCE:

I have seen more than a thousand intracellular folate deficiencies that experience a majority of these problems on the list above. A lack of folate is very common, especially those who have MTHFR. Generally, physicians rarely suspect B12 problems, or know how to treat it properly. Many times their patients find solutions at my office.

# CHAPTER THIRTEEN:
## TEN BENEFITS OF GLUTAMINE

- Helps with Short Bowel Syndrome by improving intestinal absorption.[96]

- Improves gastrointestinal health by rebuilding and repairing the intestines.[97]

- Reduces the severity of platinum induced neuropathy.[98]

- Supports and boosts immune health.[99]

- Reduces risk of cardiovascular factors substantially for those with Type 2 diabetes.[100]

- Decreases the severity of mucositis in those who underwent chemotherapy.[101]

- Helps with weight loss.[102]

- Helps maintain muscle strength, even after having surgery.[103]

- Lowers the risk of high dose chemotherapy and radiation while benefiting the overall outcome.[104]

- Improves glycemic control in those with Type 1 diabetes.[105]

- BONUS: Can help with anxiety by forming GABA.[106]

## MY MEDICAL EXPERIENCE:

Glutamine is critical to insulin receptor function and weight control; I occasionally suggest it for those issues. More importantly, I use it for certain patients with severe anxiety after performing a genetic test on them to ascertain they have a pathway error. For these patients, supplementing glutamine is important since they cannot form sufficient amounts of GABA.

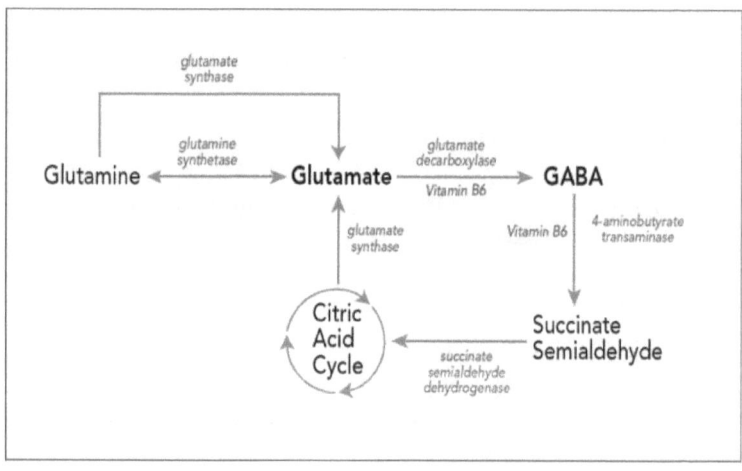

# CHAPTER FOURTEEN:
## FOUR BENEFITS OF ASPARAGINE

- Essential for protein production in the body.[107]

- Converts to aspartate providing energy in the cell (very important for those who perform manual labor or regularly workout) (see TCA Cycle).[108]

- Acts as an attachment site for carbohydrates in the cell, helping with fatigue before and after exercise.[109]

- Component in the Urea cycle helping remove excess ammonia from the body and is critical to the TCA Cycle.[110]

## MY MEDICAL EXPERIENCE:

I personally have suffered from an asparagine deficiency. I was oddly tired, could not recover from anything, and was constantly hungry. It turns out that is exactly how an asparagine deficiency would and should feel. I do not have microcephaly, hyperreflexia, or an ASNS genetic error. I do not know, nor cannot seem to find out, why I had this deficiency.

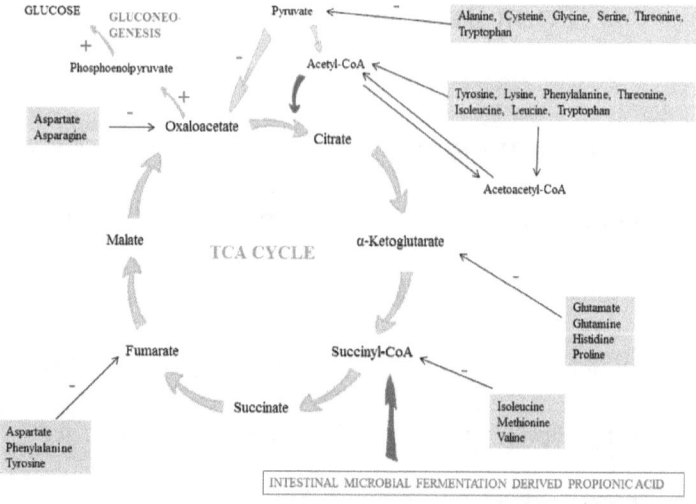

# CHAPTER FIFTEEN:
## TEN BENEFITS OF SERINE

- Improves social function in those with Autism Spectrum Disorders in the form of DCS.[111]

- Helps with weight gain in those with Anorexia Nervosa in the form of DCS.[112]

- Helps anxiety disorders and may benefit those with PTSD in the form of DCS.[113]

- Helps manage OCD in the form of DCS. [114]

- Helps manage depression in the form of DCS.[115]

- Improves brain function in adults in the form of DCS.[116]

- Helps manage Schizophrenia.[117]

- Reduces craving of alcohol in those who abuse it.[118]

- Helps with nervous system (see all the above).

- Helps the immune system create antibodies.[119]

## MY MEDICAL EXPERIENCE:

Most physicians do not know what serine is, let alone whether if it's a vitamin or an amino acid. Serine is

Vitamin B6 and critical for brain function. The worse symptoms I frequently see from serine deficiencies is depression and compulsive behavior. Usually the family brings them in on more than one antidepressant. After learning of the deficiency, we begin on serine and after about 100 days the symptoms begin to resolve. Many times they are amazed at the results, but it's just replacing a deficient vitamin.

# CHAPTER SIXTEEN:
## TEN BENEFITS OF CARNITINE

- Helps manage pain for those with Fibromyalgia.[120]

- Reduces inflammation in those who have Coronary Artery Disease.[121]

- Improves cognition in those who have Alzheimer's Disease along with other vitamins.[122]

- Prevents pancreatic cancer in those who are carnitine deficient.[123]

- Helps with Peripheral Neuropathy in those who are undergoing cancer treatment.[124]

- Helps manage depression.[125]

- Improves sperm quality in men who might be infertile.[126]

- Helps with weight loss by improving metabolism.[127]

- Helps maintain muscle strength.[128]

- Helps with erectile dysfunction.[129]

## MY MEDICAL EXPERIENCE:

Carnitine is very helpful in perceived erectile dysfunction (ED). I have young males come in with complaints that they have ED. When I learn from intracellular testing of their low testosterone and carnitine, I have them take carnitine (and usually additionally ornithine). Generally, six months later they do not have ED or low testosterone anymore.

# CHAPTER SEVENTEEN:
## TEN BENEFITS OF OLEIC ACID

- Lowers blood pressure and help with cardiovascular diseases.[130]

- Helps stop Melanoma Malignancy.[131]

- Has the potential to put out an anticancer effect.[132]

- Helps manage of esophageal cancer.[133]

- Improves glucose and insulin control.[134]

- Helps manage autoimmune diseases.[135]

- Facilitates wound healing.[136]

- Eliminates pathogens like bacteria and fungi.

- Helps with skin papilloma's while repairing skin.[137]

- Helps with inflammatory diseases especially in coronary artery disease.[138]

## MY MEDICAL EXPERIENCE:

NOTE: Oleic acid is essentially fish oil, actually being the DHA and EPA portions of the oil. DHA and EPA are the Omega-3s. You do not want the inflammatory Omega-6 oils (flax seed or even excessive olive oil). Your minimum daily dose of both should be 2,500mg total. Currently, I suggest one fish oil on the market since it only takes two large gel caps daily to almost reach 2,500mg. These gel caps are molecularly distilled and pharmaceutical grade.

I usually suggest this as TBI, or CTE, from the NFL Players Association brain trauma study is now using the high dose fish oil treatment for these brain injuries. TBI therapy requires 5,000-7,000mg (5-7 grams) of high quality DHA and EPA daily, so do not be afraid to increase daily dosage. I have seen miraculous things happen with higher doses while treating other brain injuries from motor vehicle accidents or traumatic events.

# CHAPTER EIGHTEEN:
## TEN BENEFITS OF VITAMIN D3

- Vitamin D3 deficiency increases cardiovascular risk including HOMA-IR, TC/HDL, and LDL/HDL.[139]

- Vitamin D deficiency is associated with risk of rickets in children, osteomalacia in adults, increased risk of fractures, falls, cancer, autoimmune disease, infectious disease, diabetes (Type 1 and Type 2), hypertension, heart disease, multiple sclerosis.[140]

- Has a restorative effect in knee osteoarthritis while reducing knee pain and increasing quadriceps strength.[141]

- Benefits neurological issues like Parkinson's[142] and mania in youth with bipolar spectrum disorders while improving bone health.[143]

- Inhibits the proliferation of cell growth in thyroid Cancer cells.[144]

- Helps glycemic control in children and adolescents with Type 2 diabetes, along with a significant decrease in BMI SDS, ALT, and a clinically-significant decrease in HbA1c.[145]

- Children with Type 1 diabetes generally have a significant deficiency in Vitamin D3, increasing risk for skeletal fragility and insulin resistance.[146]

- Vitamin D3 deficiency is common after TBI along with impaired cognitive function as well as those with severe depression symptoms.[147]

- Helps with chronic pain and Fibromyalgia symptoms.[148]

- Improves cardiovascular mortality, lowers rates of infections, improves glycemic indexes along with better glucose control.[149]

## MY MEDICAL EXPERIENCE:

Practicing medicine and living in Utah means that I often

prescribe 5,000-10,000mg of Vitamin D3 daily. Vitamin D3 should be taken in the morning (while calcium should be taken at night). Also, serum levels should be monitored once or twice a year to assure the Vitamin D3 does not become toxic (very uncommon). A borderline high Vitamin D3 level, called a 25(OH)D, in the 90's helps prevent two major killers, diabetes and breast cancer.

# CHAPTER NINETEEN:
## TEN BENEFITS OF RETINOL (VITAMIN A)

- Improves photodamaged skin.[150]

- Necessary for skin health.[151]

- Improves the treatment of mild cases of acne in the form of retinol and with other skin products.[152]

- Used for anti-aging and helps with wrinkles while improving skin firmness.[153]

- Reduces maternal infections while minimizing risk of anemia during pregnancy.[154]

- Essential for vision.[155]

- Essential for bone growth.[156]

- Used to prevent cancer since it can stop the proliferation of cancer cells.[157]

- Improves the immune system.[158] [159]

- Helps manage Type 2 diabetes.[160]

## MY MEDICAL EXPERIENCE:

I use tretinoin all the time in our cosmetics practice for sun damage and wrinkling. However, I have patients referred to me by ophthalmologist for night blindness. They had severe Vitamin A deficiencies on intracellular testing which surprised me since I was unaware this could happen in modern-America (like the scurvy cases I see). Be careful treating a Vitamin A deficiency as it is easy for Vitamin A levels to become toxic. Make sure to have levels checked often.

# CHAPTER TWENTY:
## TEN BENEFITS OF VITAMIN K2

- Prevents vascular calcification in hemodialysis patients.[161]

- Alternative treatment for Thalassemic Osteopathy along with Vitamin D.[162]

- Increases bone quality and prevents bone loss in postmenopausal women.[163]

- Improves bone status for those who had a lung or heart transplant.[164]

- Helps prevent liver cancer.[165]

- Helps with anemia in those with MDS when used with Vitamin D3.[166]

- Helps with osteoporosis.[167] [168]

- Helps prevent cardiovascular diseases.[169]

- Helps improve coagulation.[170]

- Acts as an anti-inflammatory.[171]

## MY MEDICAL EXPERIENCE:

I mostly use Vitamin K2 (as MK7) to reverse osteoporosis cases (usually these are bisphosphonate failures with jaw erosion problems). This approach has great success and I love seeing those who were once hopeless find a solution for their severe vitamin deficiencies.

I often prescribe ADK as well since studies have shown a better absorption of fat-soluble vitamins together than apart. I will prescribe Vitamin K2 (again as MK4) to help with bad coronary artery disease cases (CAD). Here's an ad for a MK4 I found interesting:

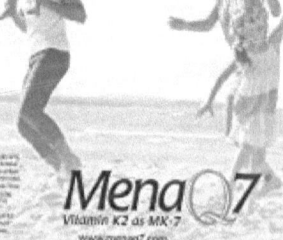

# CHAPTER TWENTY-ONE:
## TEN BENEFITS OF CALCIUM

- Lowers blood pressure in postmenopausal women.[172]

- Lowers the chance of osteoporosis in postmenopausal women.[173]

- Increases bone building in those who have osteoporosis.[174]

- Calcium carbonate helps with heartburn.[175]

- Helps with hyperphosphatemia.[176]

- Calcium Hydroxide helps improve the sealing of roots in a root canal.[177]

- Calcium in toothpaste helps with white spot lesions.[178]

- Calcium in chewing gum helps with tooth sensitivity.[179]

- Helps with bone strength in older men (like in postmenopausal women).[180]

- Helps with pregnancy-induced leg cramps.[181]

## MY MEDICAL EXPERIENCE:

I mostly use calcium like how I do Vitamin K2 to reverse osteoporosis cases (usually these are bisphosphonate failures with jaw erosion problems). This approach has great success and I love seeing those who were once hopeless find a solution for their severe vitamin deficiencies.

The minimum daily dose is 1,500mg of calcium citrate or any form besides calcium carbonate (never use since it is full of lead according to JAMA Study in 2002). Cheap forms of calcium carbonate are everywhere so be aware and avoid it.

# CHAPTER TWENTY-TWO:
## TEN BENEFITS OF MANGANESE

- ⌄ Improves bone strength and health by incorporating calcium into the bones.[182]

- ⌄ Used to help prevent osteoporosis.[183]

- ⌄ Too much manganese can lead to Parkinson-like symptoms and the disease itself.[184]

- ⌄ Helps prevent or decrease frequency of epilepsy along with other essential nutrients.[185]

- ⌄ Acts as an anti-inflammatory.[186]

- ⌄ May help prevent carcinogenesis.[187]

- ⌄ Acts as an anti-oxidant removing free radicals from the body.[188]

- ⌄ Essential for energy metabolism.[189]

- ⌄ Helps with the immune system.[190]

- ⌄ Helps with PMS symptoms.[191]

## MY MEDICAL EXPERIENCE:

This is the fourth or fifth element I prescribe for severe osteoporosis cases as it is critical to flipping these cases over the years. Manganese can be found in pineapples and can help prevent bone fractures and osteoporosis.

You may want to consider taking a high-quality manganese supplement if you are keeping to a low-carb diet and have diabetes, metabolic syndrome X, or osteoporosis. Foods such as grains, legumes, and starchy vegetables are high in manganese content, but are not allowed on low-carb diets. Blackberries, raspberries, spinach, and ginger are good sources of manganese that can be incorporated in a low-carb diet.

# CHAPTER TWENTY-THREE:
## TEN BENEFITS OF ZINC

- Lessens the effects of dysmenorrhea in young females.[192]

- Lowers the risk of complications of zinc-deficient women during pregnancy.[193]

- Helps with depression management in those who have MS.[194]

- Reduces the severity of common cold symptoms in children.[195]

- Zinc added to acne products helps the products' effectiveness.[196]

- Zinc amino acid chelate reduces respiratory infections and diarrhea in children.[197]

- Zinc oxide is an alternative way to treat warts.[198]

- Zinc oxide in ointment helps wound healing in post-surgery.[199]

⌄ Lowers the erythropoietin response in those going under hemodialysis while helping those who might have anemia.[200]

⌄ Inhibits macular degeneration.[201]

## MY MEDICAL EXPERIENCE:

After diagnosing a zinc deficiency with intracellular tests, I find that I often prescribe it when men have low testosterone or women have osteoporosis. Many 'pseudo-hypothyroid' cases are actually just zinc deficiencies (my bestselling books 'No More Cold Hands, Cold Feet' and 'Resolving Osteoporosis: The Cure & Guidebook' go into more detail on these particular cases).

J Am Coll Nutr. 2015;34(5):391-9. doi: 10.1080/07315724.2014.926161. Epub 2015 Mar 11.

**Effects of Zinc and Selenium Supplementation on Thyroid Function in Overweight and Obese Hypothyroid Female Patients: A Randomized Double-Blind Controlled Trial.**

Mahmoodianfard S[1], Vafa M[2,3], Golgiri F[3], Khoshniat M[4], Gohari M[5], Solati Z[1], Djalali M[1].

⊕ Author information

Abstract

**OBJECTIVE:** Zinc (Zn) and selenium (Se) are essential trace elements involved in thyroid hormone metabolism. This study was conducted to investigate the effects of Zn and Se supplementation on thyroid function of overweight or obese female hypothyroid patients in a double-blind, randomized controlled trial.

**METHODS:** Sixty-eight female hypothyroid patients were randomly allocated to one of the 4 supplementation groups receiving Zn + Se (ZS; 30 mg Zn as zinc-gluconate and 200 μg Se as high-selenium yeast), Zn + placebo (ZP), Se + placebo (SP), or placebo + placebo (PP) for 12 weeks. Serum Zn, Se, free and total triiodothyronine (FT3 and FT4), free and total thyroxine (FT4 and TT4), thyroid-stimulating hormone (TSH), and anthropometric parameters were measured. Dietary intake was recorded using 24-hour food recall. Physical activity questionnaire was completed.

**RESULTS:** No significant alterations were found in serum Zn or Se concentrations. Mean serum FT3 increased significantly in the ZS and ZP groups ($p < 0.05$) but this effect was significant in the ZP group compared to those in SP or PP groups ($p < 0.05$). Mean serum FT4 increased and TSH decreased significantly ($p < 0.05$) in the ZS group. TT3 and TT4 decreased significantly in the SP group ($p < 0.05$). Mean FT3:FT4 ratio was augmented significantly in the ZP group ($p < 0.05$). No significant treatment effects were found for TT3, FT4, TT4, or TSH between groups.

**CONCLUSION:** This study showed some evidence of an effect of Zn alone or in combination with Se on thyroid function of overweight or obese female hypothyroid patients.

# CHAPTER TWENTY-FOUR:
## TEN BENEFITS OF COPPER

- Helps repair photodamaged facial skin.[202]

- Copper histidine is a treatment option for Menkes disease.[203]

- Copper oxide administered topically can improve skin health.[204]

- Acts as an anti-bacterial and lowers the risk of infection.[205]

- Helps with arthritis.[206]

- Helps with premature graying hair.[207]

- Copper toxicity leads to cognition problems as well as Alzheimer's in the elderly.[208]

- Essential for normal brain growth, but excess or deficiency can cause problems such as neutropenia or anemia.[209]

- Essential for the production of thyroid, but too much or too little can cause problems.[210]

ᵛ Helps with cardiovascular health at the right

amount.[211]

## MY MEDICAL EXPERIENCE:

I have diagnosed and treated three patients with leucopenia related to copper deficiency. Their physicians were confused and unsure as how to treat their condition. I was able to treat their symptoms when I saw their low intracellular levels of copper on the SpectraCell® panel. Six months later, their white blood cell count had returned to normal.

If you have fibromyalgia (or any symptoms of fibromyalgia), you probably have a copper metallothionein dysfunction and should be treated immediately. For more information, be sure to watch my Dan Purser MD channel on YouTube that covers copper deficiencies in great detail.

J Community Hosp Intern Med Perspect. 2017 Sep 19;7(4):265-268. doi: 10.1080/20009666.2017.1351289. eCollection 2017 Oct.

**Copper deficiency, a new triad: anemia, leucopenia, and myeloneuropathy.**

Wazir SM[1], Ghobrial I[2].

⊕ Author information

Abstract

Clinical copper deficiency is now more frequently recognized. Hematologically, it can present as anemia (microcytic, normocytic, or macrocytic) and neutropenia. Thrombocytopenia is relatively rare. Neurologically, it can manifest as myelopathy and peripheral neuropathy simulating subacute combined degeneration. Bone marrow findings can mimic myelodysplasia resulting in occasional inappropriate referral for bone marrow transplantation. Other conditions with similar presentations include infections, drug toxicity, autoimmunity, $B_{12}$ deficiency, folate deficiency, myelodysplastic syndrome, aplastic anemia, and lymphoma with bone marrow involvement. Hematological, but not neurological, manifestations respond promptly to copper replacement, making early diagnosis essential for good outcome. Common risk factors for copper deficiency are foregut surgery, dietary deficiency, enteropathies with malabsorption, and prolonged intravenous nutrition (total parenteral nutrition). We present a unique case of copper deficiency, with no apparent known risk factors.

KEYWORDS: Copper; anemia; leukopenia; myelopathy

# CHAPTER TWENTY-FIVE:
## TEN BENEFITS OF MAGNESIUM

- Magnesium sulfate is an effective and fast-acting option to relieve migraines.[212]

- Intravenous Magnesium sulfate, within the first hour of hospitalization, helps those who have acute asthma without the need of mechanical ventilation support.[213]

- Magnesium sulfate can reduce the degree of fasciculation after anesthesia.[214]

- Improves the physical performance[215] in those who use it daily.[216]

- Treats pregnancy-induced leg cramps.[217]

- Adding magnesium with anesthesia helps with muscle relaxation significantly.[218]

- Helps improve respiratory muscles strength in those with cystic fibrosis.[219]

- Adding magnesium sulfate to interscalene nerve blockers prolongs the effects of feeling no pain along with lower pain levels after surgery.[220]

- Magnesium chloride applied topically helps those with fibromyalgia.[221]

- Improves the glycemic status in those who have pre-diabetes when taken orally.[222]

## MY MEDICAL EXPERIENCE:

Leg cramps are the most common symptom why I prescribe Magnesium Glycinate. These cramps can be strong enough to wake you up at night. Take enough magnesium and a few days later these cramps will improve, if not stop altogether. Do not stop taking the RDA of magnesium.

I prescribe magnesium most commonly for osteoporosis, but I rarely see anyone on it specifically for osteoporosis (but they will be on bisphosphonates with countless side effects). I track intracellular and serum levels until my osteoporosis patients do not have the deficiencies anymore.

# CHAPTER TWENTY-SIX:
## TEN BENEFITS OF CHROMIUM

- Helps moderate blood glucose levels in those with Type 2 diabetes.[223]

- Helps with food cravings.[224]

- Helps manage cholesterol.[225]

- Reduces the risk of cardiovascular disease.[226]

- Helps metabolism.[227]

- Chromium deficiency can lead to decreased fertility.[228]

- May help increase longevity of life.

- Helps with insulin resistance.[229]

- May help with neuropathy.[230]

- Chromium deficiency may lead to cardiovascular risks.[231]

## MY MEDICAL EXPERIENCE:

Chromium is critical for the insulin receptor and its functionality. I see a lot of new diabetics who are looking for help and I tell them to start exercising (mildly at first and after cardiology approval), go on low-carb diet (no easy or simple carbs!)[232], and check intracellular levels. When I perform an intracellular SpectraCell® panel, I often find a chromium deficiency and/or a zinc deficiency. By treating their deficiency problems along with their lifestyle changes, we follow serial HgbA1C until it normalizes. I warn them if they revert back to their previous lifestyle the diabetes will return with a vengeance.

# CHAPTER TWENTY-SEVEN:
## TEN BENEFITS OF GLUTATHIONE

- Helps slow Alzheimer's disease along with mild cognitive impairment.

- Delays and prevents diabetic retinopathy.

- GSH helps in the development and treatment of cancer while not undergoing chemotherapy or radiation.

- Helps with cardiovascular disease alleviating hypertension and controlling cholesterol.

- Acts as an anti-inflammatory.

- Helps in the treatment of cystic fibrosis.

- Improves the immune system and fights infections.

- Helps in the treatment of diabetes.

- Helps with acne.

- Slows and prevents age-related complications.

- Reduces oxidative stress.

## MY MEDICAL EXPERIENCE:

Glutathione is a hot topic nationwide. We have developed and patented the only functional (validated, absorbable, reduced and stable) glutathione or GSH on the market today. We have not found a functional, working, reduced, or validated glutathione on the market (despite the 50+ products we have bought and tested). If you are deficient in glutathione on your intracellular testing, suffer from brain fog, or experience fatigue, you should get a bottle of VARS Mint Burst Glutathione and try it orally.

You should know that if your glutathione level is low it almost is assured that your homocysteine level is high which is very bad. You need address your MTHFR problems and I suggest getting genetic testing. If your MTHFR is confirmed, you should try our MTHFR Support or MTHFR Support Plus products. I always suggest starting low and go up slowly. For more information, be sure to check out my bestselling book 'The 85% Solution' on Amazon.

# CHAPTER TWENTY-EIGHT:
## TEN BENEFITS OF CYSTEINE

- Lowers homocysteine levels and lowers blood pressure which helps prevent vascular events in the form of N-Acetylcysteine (NAC).[233]

- Helps elderly increase muscle strength when added to protein powder.[234]

- Helps prevent strokes.[235]

- Alternative treatment as NAC to help those with autistic disorders.[236]

- Helps reduce oxidative stress.[237]

- Maintains lung function in those with Cystic Fibrosis.[238]

- Helps prevent Nonthyroidal Illness Syndrome.[239]

- May help with neurological disorders.[240 241]

- Increases glutathione levels.[242]

- Improves fertility in women with PCOS.[243]

## MY MEDICAL EXPERIENCE:

I generally use cysteine, or NAC, when there is a deficiency on intracellular tests. A cysteine deficiency is usually associated with MTHFR, so I usually address that as well.

# CHAPTER TWENTY-NINE:
## TEN BENEFITS OF CoQ10 (UBIQUINOL)

- Those who have a hard time on statins for dyslipidemia, CoQ10 can be a substitute, along with other nutraceuticals, for the same effect and gentler on the body (CoQ10 can also be used with the statin).[244]

- Reduces statin myopathy symptoms.[245]

- Helps those with Chronic Heart Failure when used long-term, while improving symptoms and reducing major adverse cardiovascular events.[246]

- Improves health and heart function for those with Congestive Heart Failure.[247]

- Alternate treatment method to treat hypertension.[248]

- Helps children with autism.[249]

- Helps with ovulation and increases pregnancy rate for women with PCOS when used along with Clomiphene Citrate.[250]

- Reduces the frequency of migraines and headaches.[251]

- Improves the survival rate for those with end-stage cancer.[252]

- Those with breast cancer are able to see a partial, or full regression, of their tumors.[253]

## MY MEDICAL EXPERIENCE:

Ubiquinol is the only coenzyme that participates in both the citric acid cycle (TCA) and the electron transport chain. In Step 8 of the citric acid cycle, SQR catalyzes the oxidation of succinate to fumarate with the reduction of ubiquinone to ubiquinol. Ubiquinol is nine times more absorbable than ubiquinone.

The primary reason I prescribe ubiquinol is if the patient currently takes thyroid medication. If they take thyroid hormone, they should take 200mg+ daily to offset the forced loss in the Krebs Cycle and TCA. If you are suffering from brain fog, or experiencing fatigue, you should get a bottle of VARS Mint Burst Glutathione and try it orally.

# Krebs Cycle Nutrients

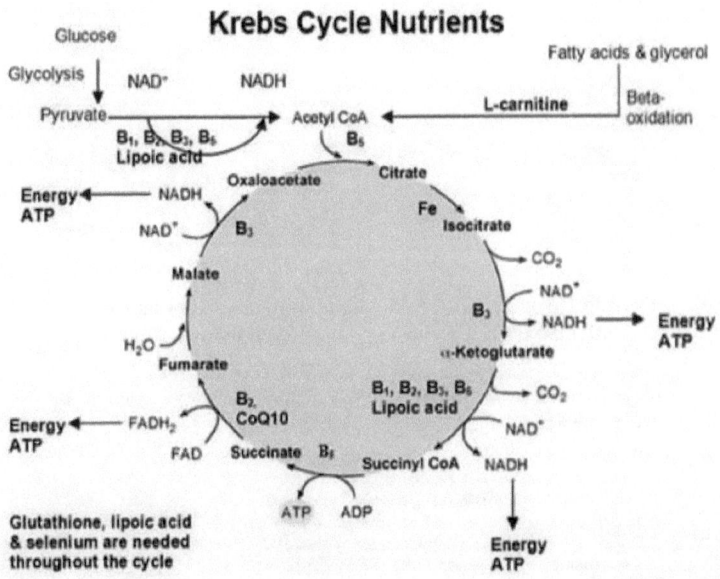

*Int. J. Mol. Sci.* **2013**, *14*, 23893-23909; doi:10.3390/ijms141223893

OPEN ACCESS

International Journal of
**Molecular Sciences**
ISSN 1422-0067
www.mdpi.com/journal/ijms

*Review*

# Thyroid Hormones and Antioxidant Systems: Focus on Oxidative Stress in Cardiovascular and Pulmonary Diseases

**Antonio Mancini** [1,*], **Sebastiano Raimondo** [1], **Chantal Di Segni** [1], **Mariasara Persano** [1], **Giovanni Gadotti** [1], **Andrea Silvestrini** [2], **Roberto Festa** [3], **Luca Tiano** [4], **Alfredo Pontecorvi** [1] and **Elisabetta Meucci** [2]

[1] Department of Medical Sciences, Division of Endocrinology, Catholic University;
Rome 00168, Italy; E-Mails: bastio984@hotmail.com (S.R.);
chantal_ds86@hotmail.com (C.D.S.); sarapers@hotmail.it (M.P.);
giovanni.gadotti@gmail.com (G.G.); pontecorvi@rm.unicatt.it (A.P.)

[2] Institute of Biochemistry and Clinical Biochemistry, Catholic University, Rome 00168, Italy;
E-Mails: asilvestrini@rm.unicatt.it (A.S.); emeucci@rm.unicatt.it (E.M.)

[3] Department of Clinical and Molecular Science, Polytechnic University of the Marche,
Ancona 60100, Italy, E-Mail: festa7r@libero.it

[4] Department of Clinical and Dental Sciences, Polytechnic University of Marche, Ancona 60100, Italy;
E-Mail: l.tiano@univpm.it

* Author to whom correspondence should be addressed; E-Mail: mancini.giac@mclink.it;
Tel.: +39-06-3015-4440; Fax: +39-06-3015-7232.

*Received: 18 September 2013; in revised form: 11 November 2013 / Accepted: 21 November 2013 / Published: 9 December 2013*

**Abstract:** In previous works we demonstrated an inverse correlation between plasma Coenzyme $Q_{10}$ ($CoQ_{10}$) and thyroid hormones; in fact, $CoQ_{10}$ levels in hyperthyroid patients were found among the lowest detected in human diseases. On the contrary, $CoQ_{10}$ is elevated in hypothyroid subjects, also in subclinical conditions, suggesting the usefulness of this index in assessing metabolic status in thyroid disorders. A Low-T3 syndrome is a condition observed in several chronic diseases: it is considered an adaptation mechanism, where there is a reduction in pro-hormone T4 conversion. Low T3-Syndrome is not usually considered to be corrected with replacement therapy. We review the role of thyroid hormones in regulation of antioxidant systems, also presenting data on total antioxidant capacity and Coenzyme $Q_{10}$. Published studies suggest that oxidative stress could be involved in the clinical course of different heart diseases; our data could support the rationale of replacement therapy in low-T3 conditions.

# CHAPTER THIRTY:
## TEN BENEFITS OF SELENIUM

- Helps improve glucose control for those with diabetes.[254]

- Reduces the side effects of chemotherapy.[255]

- Improves the treatment of Chagas cardiopathy.[256]

- Has an anti-inflammatory [257] and an anti-viral effect.

- Selenium deficiency has been linked to rheumatoid arthritis.[258]

- May prevent cancer, especially prostate cancer, when used along with Vitamin E.[259]

- Helps prevent sunburns when used along with other antioxidants.[260]

- Helps with thyroid autoimmune disorders[261] and Type 2 diabetes.[262]

- Helps improve semen quality in men with fertility issues when used with Vitamin E.[263]

- Helps with neurological disorders.[264]

## MY MEDICAL EXPERIENCE:

Selenium is critical to thyroid manufacture, ATP manufacture (energy), and thyroid receptor functionality. You never want to be low in selenium. Before starting treatment to help the thyroid function, I try selenium first to correct the thyroid condition.

# CHAPTER THIRTY-ONE:
## TEN BENEFITS OF VITAMIN E (MIXED α-TOCOPHEROLS)

- Helps with daily fatigue.[265]

- Relieves symptoms of urinary tract infections in girls with pyelonephritis.[266]

- Vitamin E, as A-tocopherol, deficiency increases the risk of miscarriage.[267]

- Helps with healing photodamaged skin.[268]

- Improves cognition for those with Alzheimer's when used with essential vitamins.[269]

- Supportive therapy for Hepatitis C.[270]

- Supplemental therapy for PMS when used with Vitamin D.[271]

- Helps with arthritis.[272]

- Helps prevent cancer as an antioxidant.[273]

- Helps with aging.[274]

## MY MEDICAL EXPERIENCE:

I will give Vitamin E (as Mixed $\alpha$-Tocopherols) to patients who have genetic conditions or intracellular levels requiring it. A few say they felt amazing when taking it, which I thought was unusual, but they had severe deficiencies.

# CHAPTER THIRTY-TWO:
## TEN BENEFITS OF ALPHA LIPOIC ACID

- Significantly helps Endothelial dysfunction for adolescents with Type 1 diabetes when used with an antioxidant diet.[275]

- Helps with male infertility.[276]

- Helps with Peripheral Neuropathy for those with diabetes.[277]

- Improves insulin control in those who are diabetic.[278]

- Exerts a neuroprotective effect by reducing oxidative stress.[279]

- Helps with hypertension.[280]

- Improves glutathione levels in the body.[281]

- Helps with anti-aging and improves photodamaged skin.[282]

- Removes free radicals from the body when used with other antioxidants.[283]

- Helps prevent cancer and infectious diseases.[284]

## MY MEDICAL EXPERIENCE:

I usually give Alpha Lipoic Acid (600mg daily) for only three reasons: (1) deficiency on intracellular levels, (2) neuropathy in diabetic patients (I have seen a few 'miracles' from this approach), and (3) patients taking glutathione to help convert the glutathione from an oxidized state to a reduced, or active, state (GSH).

European Review for Medical and Pharmacological Sciences

2018; 22: 4739-4754

# Natural products – alpha-lipoic acid and acetyl-L-carnitine – in the treatment of chemotherapy-induced peripheral neuropathy

S. DINICOLA[1,2], A. FUSO[2,3], A. CUCINA[3,4], M. SANTIAGO-REYES[3,4],
R. VERNA[1,2], V. UNFER[5], G. MONASTRA[2], M. BIZZARRI[1,2]

[1]Department of Experimental Medicine, Sapienza University of Rome, Rome, Italy
[2]Systems Biology Group Lab, Sapienza University of Rome, Rome, Italy
[3]Department of Surgery "Pietro Valdoni", Sapienza University of Rome, Rome, Italy
[4]Azienda Policlinico Umberto I, Rome, Italy
[5]Department of Developmental and Social Psychology, Faculty of Medicine and Psychology,
Sapienza University of Rome, Rome, Italy

**Abstract.** – OBJECTIVE: Cancer patients frequently experience Chemotherapy-Induced Peripheral Neuropathy (CIPN), as a typical side effect related to time of administration and dose of anticancer agents. Yet, CIPN pathophysiology is poorly understood, and there is a lack of well-tolerated pharmacological remedies helpful to prevent or treat it. Therefore, new safe and effective compounds are highly warranted, namely if based on an adequate understanding of the pathogenic mechanisms.
MATERIAL AND METHODS: Herein we reviewed and discussed scientific data related to the beneficial role of some non-conventional treatments able to counteract CIPN, focusing our attention on alpha-lipoic acid (ALA) and L-acetyl-carnitine (LAC), two natural products that have been demonstrated to be promising preventive drugs.
RESULTS: Although a growing body of in vitro and in vivo studies support ALA as a molecule able to counteract CIPN symptoms, mostly due to its antioxidant and anti-inflammatory properties, only two randomized clinical trials evaluated ALA usefulness in preventing chemotherapy-related neuropathy. Unfortunately, these studies were inconclusive and clinical outcomes showed to be highly dependent on the route of administration (oral versus or intravenous injection). LAC has demonstrated beneficial effects on both in vitro and in animal studies. Yet, some controversies aroused from randomized clinical trials. Indeed, while CIPN-patients treated with Taxane showed no benefit from LAC treatment, CIPN-patients treated with platinum compounds exhibit significant improvement of CIPN-related symptoms. Therefore, LAC treatment should be used, and thoroughly investigated only in patients treated with chemotherapy protocols Taxanes-free.

CONCLUSIONS: Mechanisms of toxicity triggered by each single drug need to be deeply explored to better identify effective compounds to prevent or treat them. Moreover, additional experiments are mandatory to establish effective doses and length of treatment for each clinical situation in order to perform large and long-term randomized studies.

Key Words:
Alpha-Lipoic acid, Acetyl-L-Carnitine, Chemotherapy, Peripheral Neuropathy.

## Introduction

Chemotherapy (CT)-Induced Peripheral Neuropathy (CIPN) is a frequent and potentially debilitating side effect of cancer treatment. Peripheral neuropathy, manifested by neuropathic pain and axonal degeneration, is indeed one of the major sources of disability in patients following antineoplastic therapy after hematological and renal toxicity[1,2]. Availability of efficient anti-emetic drugs and hematopoietic colony stimulating factors has allowed in the last decades high-dosage CT regimens, especially those including 'aggressive' antineoplastic drugs. Consequently, serious side effects including CIPN are currently more frequently observed than in the past and often represent a dose-limiting factor in treatment delivery. Despite its clinical relevance and common occurrence, the epidemiology as well as the pathophysiology of CIPN in the different groups of chemotherapies is still

Corresponding Author: Simona Dinicola, Ph.D; e-mail: simona.dinicola@uniroma1.it

# CHAPTER THIRTY-THREE:
## TEN BENEFITS OF VITAMIN C

- Alternative option to handle anxiety.[285]

- Lowers frequency of the common cold.[286]

- Manages Complex Regional Pain Syndrome Type I (in wrists and ankles) after surgery.[287]

- Lessens recovery time of burn wounds when used along with Vitamin E and Zinc.[288]

- May help in removing dark circles under eyes.[289]

- Helps skin recover from sun damage when topically applied and used with madecassoside.[290]

- Using intravenous Vitamin C during chemotherapy increases the effectiveness of the chemotherapy.[291]

- Helps prevent and manage Upper Respiratory Tract Infections in children when used with probiotics.[292]

- Helps postmenopausal women with wrinkles when used with other vitamins.[293]

˅   Helps prevent Premature Rupture of the

Chorioamniotic Membranes.[294]

## MY MEDICAL EXPERIENCE:

I have given Vitamin C clinically when severe deficiencies occur three times. This is a disease called scurvy and all three had it (one was near death). Unfortunately, other physicians were unable to make the diagnosis as they were suffering from bleeding gums, tooth loss, mouth sores, hair loss, muscle wasting, fatigue, and weakness. By addressing their vitamin deficiency, their symptoms were gone after 90 days.

# CHAPTER THIRTY-FOUR:
## PARTICULAR PROBLEMS CAUSED BY VITAMIN DEFICIENCIES

I wanted to save these until the end in case you missed my comments or studies relating to the problems. I would also like to share what I've seen in the last fifteen years of experience as I test and treat patients. I will only use one or two references per example, but there are numerous other cases I could list.

## Deficiencies Caused by Keto or Low-Carb Diets

Many people who have done great with their ketogenic or low-carb (i.e. Atkins®) feel fatigued, exhausted, and almost collapse every day. They feel tired because they have accidentally malnourished themselves during months on a low carb diet.[295] [296] This happens more often than you may think since there is no way anyone can eat perfectly. I have never tested anyone the first time and not found a deficiency. The stricter a diet is, the more deficiencies I usually find. It never surprises me when a new patient has post-diet fatigue, which is why I would advise patients interested in a particular diet to do this test before and after starting. It can save their time, energy, and health.

## Diabetes Due to Vitamin Deficiency[297]

When new diabetics (usually Type 2 diabetics) come in, they want a more natural approach to their diabetes. From a SpectraCell® Micronutrient Panel, I usually find a zinc or chromium deficiency (among many other deficiencies). Usually, if their diagnosis is recent, we treat all their vitamin deficiencies, get them walking (1-4-7)*, lifting mild weights (three times weekly), and stopping all carbs for three months. I see a high success rate in 'flipping' them out of their diabetes if they follow these recommendations diligently. This is definitely better than needing to take diabetic medications for the rest of their lives.

*1-4-7 comes from my Program120 Textbook on Preventative Medicine meaning walking one hour daily, walking four miles per hour, seven days a week.

## Low Testosterone Due to Vitamin Deficiency[298]

From my endocrinology research and bestselling book on men's testosterone ('Improving Male Sexuality, Fertility, and Testosterone'), many young men come into my practice with complaints of low testosterone. Instead of giving them testosterone, I test their vitamin levels at an intracellular level. Generally, they always have B12, folate, zinc, serine, carnitine, and other deficiencies (granted almost everyone in Utah comes from northern European descent consisting of blonde hair, blue eyes, and MTHFR). Initially, they are usually surprised when I do not prescribe them testosterone. However, once identifying and treating their deficiencies, most have normal levels of testosterone after six to nine months. This process takes a little longer, but these men are not temporarily sterilized from testosterone prescriptions other physicians would prescribe.

## Fatigue and Vitamin Deficiency[299]

Throughout this book, we have covered fatigue is the primary symptom of vitamin deficiencies. It is the body sending a warning signal that something is wrong. I rarely, if ever, prescribe any amphetamine because I am looking for the root cause. By doing so, I am able to help most of my patients get off their amphetamines for fatigue that other physicians prescribe immediately. Be sure to watch my videos on my YouTube channel ('Dan Purser MD') for more information on fatigue.

## Anxiety and Depression Caused by Vitamin Deficiency[300]

After all these years and thousands of patients, I believe the most common cause of depression is a genetic error causing a vitamin deficiency (especially B vitamins).[301] If you're on antidepressant or antianxiety medications, I would definitely recommend learning what is happening through a SpectraCell® Micronutrient Panel and genetic testing.

## Infertility Due to Vitamin Deficiency

Throughout the years, I have sat across from hundreds of crying, exhausted female patients (along with their husbands) facing infertility. Majority of these infertility cases, both male and female, are due to vitamin deficiencies (particularly B vitamin deficiencies) and genetic errors. In Utah, these cases tend to come from either MTHFR or a Vitamin D deficiency [302] due to longer winters. I have also found severe post-partum fatigue/exhaustion/depression is almost always caused by major genetics-related vitamin deficiencies. As I mentioned before, if you're on an antidepressant, I would definitely recommend learning what is happening through a SpectraCell® Micronutrient Panel and genetic testing.

## Neuropathy Caused by Vitamin Deficiency

From my experience, I have found B12 (methylcobalamin & hydroxocobalamin, not cyanocobalamin) and Alpha Lipoic Acid are the most common cause of vitamin deficiencies resulting in any type of neuropathy.[303] I deal with this frequently and have seen so many patients suffer from this pain for years. It is amazing what natural B12 shots can do (not cyanocobalamin shots, you must get it compounded). If you are suffering from any type of neuropathy, I would definitely recommend learning what is happening through a SpectraCell® Micronutrient Panel and genetic testing.

## Women's Hair Loss and Vitamin Deficiency[304]

I would recommend reading Spencer David Kobren's bestselling book 'The Bald Truth About Women's Hair Loss'. I agree with Spencer that the most common cause of women's hair loss is a vitamin deficiency (especially B vitamins). If you have unexplained hair loss, I would definitely recommend learning what is happening through a SpectraCell® Micronutrient Panel and genetic testing.

## Osteoporosis and Vitamin Deficiency[305]

If you have osteoporosis (or osteopenia), check first for a vitamin deficiency. I have seen so many women (and a few men) who have horrible Vitamin D, K2, calcium, magnesium, and or zinc deficiencies suffer from symptoms of osteoporosis. Sadly, many of them were given bisphosphonates (with side effect rates of 75%) before coming to my practice. I find that absurd! My long-time friend, who was US Assistant Surgeon General, would say, "A lot of doctors are not doing their jobs!" He could not be more correct. If you're on an antidepressant, I would definitely recommend learning what is happening through a SpectraCell® Micronutrient Panel and genetic testing. For more information on osteoporosis, my bestselling book 'Resolving Osteoporosis' goes into greater depth.

# CHAPTER THIRTY-FIVE:
## PATIENT STORIES INVOLVING VITAMIN DEFICIENCIES

## A YOUNG MAN WITH LOW TESOSTERONE AND FATIGUE

He sat across from me with his wife exhausted and fatigued. He was receiving testosterone shots (testosterone cypionate) from his local doctor once every two weeks. His fatigue, which should have been resolved, had not improved. He had developed minimal interest in sex as a newlywed and his young wife was not happy.

I looked at him concerned and asked, "What did your doctor say was the cause of your low testosterone?" Both of their heads shot up with surprised looks on their faces. "He never said. I never thought to ask."

I nodded. His wife looked exasperated and they looked at each other. "How low was your first testosterone level?" I asked. His wife opened a manila file folder and pulled out the lab results, sliding it forward. I looked over the numbers. "This is treated. It's 1,067. Good number. When was this done? How many days after one of your shots?" He looked at the date and responded, "Four days."

"Are you feeling pretty good then?" I probed. He responded dejectedly, "Kind of," his wife added, "But he got really depressed and tired after about day five or six." I nodded, "I usually give them every seven days and let the patient give his own since it can be fairly expensive." They nodded.

"That way you don't have drop off." They nodded again, realization dawning. "But I'm not sure you even need testosterone – at least not for the long run."

"Why?"

"Well, we don't know the cause of your low testosterone. Did you play football or have car wreck?" They both shook their heads no. He said, "I played in the marching band in college."

I nodded. "Have you ever had a loss of consciousness event? Were you ever knocked out?" She looked at him as he thought. He finally said, "No, not ever." They both shook their heads.

I said, "I give your doctor credit for making the diagnoses, but he should have explored further. However, most don't even know to do so." They nodded.

I then told them, "I think it's nutritional, probably vitamin deficiencies. And if you have these deficiencies, they could be because your absorption of some key vitamins is blocked at a cellular level due to genetic errors passed down through your family history."

"Genetic errors?"

"Errors are usually from mutations that happened generations ago – like many hundreds of generations. What's your heritage?" He thought for a second. "My mom says we're Norwegian."

I nodded. "The only way we can tell intracellular deficiencies is through a SpectraCell® Micronutrient Panel. This is critical to move this pathway forward." His wife said, "We want to understand fully what is happening. Let's do all of the tests you suggest so we get the full picture."

"I would recommend re-testing your testosterone levels and a few pituitary labs just to make sure."

## Three Weeks Later

As we started our follow-up consultation, I handed them copies of his labs. They looked them over while I explained, "Your testosterone was low at 178 and your pituitary labs are 'lowish' as well. However, these levels lead me to think this is a malnutrition issue which is reflected in your vitamin panel."

They looked at the SpectraCell® Micronutrient Panel results. "What does this mean?" his wife asked. Her husband just looked exhausted and unmotivated.

"He has a B12, folate, pantothenate and choline deficiency – all B vitamins. And his zinc and carnitine levels are also low. If we were to check, he should have low testosterone, low libido, and low thyroid." He looked up, "Do you need to?"

"No, we don't need to check since we already know they would be low. You're malnourished, but it looks like you have a genetic error called MTHFR."

He suddenly looked excited, "My mom told me a few days ago that she and her brothers had MTHFR. She wondered if it might be my problem."

"I am guessing it is." His wife leaned forward. "So, what do we do now?"

"We treat these vitamin deficiencies with an MTHFR support type product and perform some inexpensive genetic testing to confirm what exactly you have. After three to six months, you should start to see a big rise in your hormones, especially your testosterone levels."

"So, I don't need testosterone shots?"

"Or creams or gels?" his wife added.

"We can if you're suffering, but I'd prefer to treat you this way. I've seen it work with hundreds of other patients. It should help you and you should have normal levels in a year."

"How long do I have to take the vitamins?"

"They won't cure your genetic errors. So forever… once you dial in what works." They nodded, thinking.

"Better than shots for life." They smiled knowing they found a solution for him.

## A RECENTLY DIAGNOSED FEMALE DIABETIC PATIENT

She was 43-years-old and just diagnosed with Type 2 diabetes. She began, "I heard that you have cleared up a few cases of new onset diabetes."

"Sure," I said, smiling. "It's always worth a try. What was your hemoglobin A1C when they checked it?" She responded, "6.5 and my physician told me to cut back on my carbs while increasing my exercise level. He said we would re-evaluate my levels in three months. If we don't see improvement, we may try metformin."

"That's a good plan, but we can do a lot better though. Have you been tired lately?" As she sighed, "All the time and I have gained 40 lbs."

"Do you have regular periods? Do you experience hot flashes or night sweats?" She looked at me, "Still regular. Never."

"Let's look at your vitamins first since nutrition is critical for insulin receptor functionality. If you have a zinc or chromium, your insulin receptors won't work well, if at all.

If we fix these deficiencies, the diabetes may just go away. Follow your physician's advice of reducing carbs and exercising more. However, intermittent fasting at night can also improve your insulin receptor function and cause weight loss."

"What exactly is intermittent fasting?"

"Intermittent fasting allows your body to slow the production of insulin required when eating. You simply do not eat for sixteen hours daily (i.e. 8pm to noon). Eating schedules can vary to accommodate different lifestyles and events. During these fasts, you should drink plenty of water to remain hydrated. But first let's get a SpectraCell® Micronutrient Panel for you to understand what exactly is happening."

"Can I just start on chromium now?"

"Absolutely and probably on zinc as well. I would recommend one of chromium picolinate and zinc picolinate daily." I slid some bottles forward.

**Three Weeks Later**

"So far I've lost 12 lbs. and I feel so much better. Cutting out the carbs and starting the intermittent fast was hard for the first week, but has become easier."

"That is great to hear! Keep it up and we'll continue to see results. Here is your SpectraCell® results. Looks like we were right a few weeks ago."

She looked at the panel results, "You were right, does this say I have deficiencies of chromium, zinc, B6, and glutathione?"

"Yep," I slid more bottles forward, "Reduced glutathione can definitely improve insulin receptor function. We have our VARS® Mint Burst Glutathione." I slid studies from PubMed over and said, "Here are studies validating everything we have covered today."

She leafed through them. "I'm excited there is a solution! I would have never guessed these deficiencies could have such an impact. Thank you!"

"Let's see what your A1C shows in 100 days since it usually takes that long to really change intracellular levels." She nodded and smiled.


## YOUNG WOMEN WITH 'PSEUDO-HYPOTHYROIDISM'

She stopped me as I was heading into my office, "Dr. Purser, my doctor said I was hypothyroid. Can you help me?" I looked at her, "Sure, let me feel your hands." I carefully held them. Both were ice cold in the middle of August.

"What exactly did your doctor tell you?" I asked. "He said my TSH was kind of high. Barely, but he said I needed just a tiny amount of thyroid to supplement it."

"You can't just barely treat thyroid problems. Once you start taking any oral supplement, even a tiny amount, it will suppress your own production. Either it's a lot of thyroid replacement or none." She nodded, looking concerned. I continued, "Do you have any family history of thyroid problems?"

"No."

"Have you been tired a lot?"

"Yes."

"Make sense because fatigue usually is associated with hypothyroidism. Do you have any thyroid antibodies?"

"No."

"Do you want me to make sure it's not a vitamin deficiency? It could be a zinc or selenium deficiency, or both. These deficiencies would affect your production and thyroid receptors."

"I've heard that when these deficiencies are resolved, thyroid disease is cured as well."

"Well, a decrease in thyroid hormone is generally just a symptom a symptom of a vitamin deficiency. Good nutrition going in equals good hormones coming out. Vice versa for poor nutrition and poor hormones. We should get a SpectraCell® Micronutrient Panel to look at your intracellular vitamins, minerals, and amino acids."

## Three Weeks Later

"Your SpectraCell® results show bad deficiencies of selenium and zinc along with a few others. There's your 'cure' for hypothyroidism."

"So, I don't have hypothyroidism?"

"Well, not in the autoimmune sense. Just a symptom, or side effect, of a few vitamin deficiencies."

"My doctor wanted to start me on thyroid. I could have taken that the rest of my life and not known, right?"

"Right, but he was doing the best he could. Fortunately, finding the root causes of these symptoms can resolve these problems better."

She said, "I like this way best." I smiled and handed her some vitamins, "So do I."

# FINAL THOUGHTS

Vitamin deficiencies are very real and affect thousands of people worldwide. Having just one deficiency on your SpectraCell® Micronutrient Panel can make you feel unwell, fatigued, 'brain-fogged', exhausted, depressed, anxious, or miserable.

If you have any of these symptoms we have covered throughout this book, I would recommend getting your intracellular levels tested. It's the most basic root test for health and everyone should have it performed every few years. It cannot be simpler than using vitamins to resolve seemingly complex symptoms. Usually it takes about two to three weeks for results, which can be lifechanging.

Call my office at (801) 796-7667 and mention this book to receive a 10% discount on your tests. Together we can find a solution that will help you feel better. Thank you for reading.

God bless and go in good health,

Dan Purser MD & Jared Larkin

[1] Hosseinlou A, Alinejad V, et al. The effects of fish oil capsules and vitamin B1 tablets on duration and severity of dysmenorrhea in students of high school in Urmia-Iran. Glob J Health Sci. 2014 Sep 18;6(7 Spec No):124-9. doi: 10.5539/gjhs.v6n7p124.

[2] Abdollahifard S, Rahmanian et al. The effects of vitamin B1 on ameliorating the premenstrual syndrome symptoms. Glob J Health Sci. 2014 Jul 29;6(6):144-53. doi: 10.5539/gjhs.v6n6p144.

[3] Xu G, Lv ZW, Xu GX, Tang WZ. Thiamine, cobalamin, locally injected alone or combination for herpetic itching: a single-center randomized controlled trial. Clin J Pain. 2014 Mar;30(3):269-78. doi: 10.1097/AJP.0b013e3182a0e085.

[4] Alaei Shahmiri F, Soares MJ, Zhao Y, Sherriff J. High-dose thiamine supplementation improves glucose tolerance in hyperglycemic individuals: a randomized, double-blind cross-over trial. Eur J Nutr. 2013 Oct;52(7):1821-4. doi: 10.1007/s00394-013-0534-6. Epub 2013 May 29.

[5] Schoenenberger AW, Schoenenberger-Berzins R, der Maur CA, Suter PM, Vergopoulos A, Erne P. Thiamine supplementation in symptomatic chronic heart failure: a randomized, double-blind, placebo-controlled, cross-over pilot study. Clin Res Cardiol. 2012 Mar;101(3):159-64. doi: 10.1007/s00392-011-0376-2. Epub 2011 Nov 5.

[6] Manzardo AM, Pendleton T, Poje A, Penick EC, Butler MG. Change in psychiatric symptomatology after benfotiamine treatment in males is related to lifetime alcoholism severity. Drug Alcohol Depend. 2015 Jul 1;152:257-63. doi: 10.1016/j.drugalcdep.2015.03.032. Epub 2015 Apr 8.

[7] Sugimori N, Espinoza JL, Trung LQ, Takami A, Kondo Y, An DT, Sasaki M, Wakayama T, Nakao S. Paraptosis cell death induction by the thiamine analog benfotiamine in leukemia cells. PLoS One. 2015 Apr 7;10(4):e0120709. doi: 10.1371/journal.pone.0120709. eCollection 2015.

[8] Hanberry BS, Berger R, Zastre JA. High-dose vitamin B1 reduces proliferation in cancer cell lines analogous to dichloroacetate. Cancer Chemother Pharmacol. 2014 Mar;73(3):585-94. doi: 10.1007/s00280-014-2386-z. Epub 2014 Jan 23.

[9] Lu'o'ng Kv, Nguyen LT. Role of thiamine in Alzheimer's disease. Am J Alzheimers Dis Other Demen. 2011 Dec;26(8):588-98. doi: 10.1177/1533317511432736. Epub 2012 Jan 4.

[10] Bubko I, Gruber BM, Anuszewska EL. [The role of thiamine in neurodegenerative diseases].
[Article in Polish] Postepy Hig Med Dosw (Online). 2015 Sep 21;69:1096-106.

[11] Bubko I, Gruber BM, Anuszewska EL. [The role of thiamine in neurodegenerative diseases].
[Article in Polish] Postepy Hig Med Dosw (Online). 2015 Sep 21;69:1096-106.

[12] Gaul C, Diener HC, Danesch U; Migravent® Study Group. Improvement of migraine symptoms with a proprietary supplement containing riboflavin, magnesium and Q10: a randomized, placebo-controlled, double-blind, multicenter trial. J Headache Pain. 2015;16:516. doi: 10.1186/s10194-015-0516-6. Epub 2015 Apr 3.

[13] Chutko LS, Surushkina SY, Yakovenko EA, Rozhkova AV, Anisimova TI, Bondarchuk YL. [The efficacy of cytoflavin in the treatment of burnout syndrome]. [Article in Russian] Zh Nevrol Psikhiatr Im S S Korsakova. 2015;115(10):66-70.

[14] Shen K, Huang XE. Clinical investigation in effect of riboflavin sodium phosphate on prevention and treatment for patients with radiotherapy related esophagitis. Asian Pac J Cancer Prev. 2015;16(4):1525-7.

[15] Chaves Neto AH, Pelizzaro-Rocha KJ, Fernandes MN, Ferreira-Halder CV. Antitumor activity of irradiated riboflavin on human renal carcinoma cell line 786-O. Tumour Biol. 2015 Feb;36(2):595-604. doi: 10.1007/s13277-014-2675-5. Epub 2014 Oct 2.

[16] Shi Z, Zhen S, Wittert GA, Yuan B, Zuo H, Taylor AW. Inadequate riboflavin intake and anemia risk in a Chinese population: five-year follow up of the Jiangsu Nutrition Study. PLoS One. 2014 Feb 12;9(2):e88862. doi: 10.1371/journal.pone.0088862. eCollection 2014.

[17] Tavares NR, Moreira PA, Amaral TF. Riboflavin supplementation and biomarkers of cardiovascular disease in the elderly. J Nutr Health Aging. 2009 May;13(5):441-6.

[18] Hashemi H, Seyedian MA, Miraftab M, Bahrmandy H, Sabzevari A, Asgari S. Clinical results with two different pharmaceutical preparations of riboflavin in corneal cross-linking: an 18-month follow up. Daru. 2015 Jan 24;23:4. doi: 10.1186/s40199-015-0091-z.

[19] Maisch T, Eichner A, Späth A, Gollmer A, König B, Regensburger J, Bäumler W. Fast and effective photodynamic inactivation of multiresistant bacteria by cationic riboflavin derivatives. PLoS One. 2014 Dec 3;9(12):e111792. doi: 10.1371/journal.pone.0111792. eCollection 2014.

[20] Machado D, Shishido SM, Queiroz KC, Oliveira DN, Faria AL, Catharino RR, Spek CA, Ferreira CV. Irradiated riboflavin diminishes the aggressiveness of melanoma in vitro and in vivo. PLoS One. 2013;8(1):e54269. doi: 10.1371/journal.pone.0054269. Epub 2013 Jan 16.

[21] Cheung IM, McGhee CN, Sherwin T. Beneficial effect of the antioxidant riboflavin on gene expression of extracellular matrix elements, antioxidants and oxidases keratoconic stromal cells. Clin Exp Optom. 2014 Jul;97(4):349-55. doi: 10.1111/cxo.12138. Epub 2014 Feb 17.

[22] Hamoud, Shadi, Tony Hayek, Ahmad Hassan, Edna Meilin, Marielle Kaplan, Rafael Torgovicky, and Raanan Cohen. "Niacin Administration Significantly Reduces Oxidative Stress in Patients With Hypercholesterolemia and Low Levels of High-Density Lipoprotein Cholesterol." *The American Journal of the Medical Sciences* 345, no. 3 (2013): 195-99. doi:10.1097/maj.0b013e3182548c28.

[23] Mitchel, Yale, Harold E. Bays, Eliot A. Brinton, Joseph Triscari, Erluo Chen, Darbie Maccubbin, Alexandra A. Maclean, Kendra Gibson, Rae Ann Ruck, Amy O. Johnson-Levonas, and Edward A. O'neill. "Extended-release Niacin/laropiprant Significantly Improves Lipid Levels in Type 2 Diabetes Mellitus Irrespective of Baseline Glycemic Control." *VHRM Vascular Health and Risk Management*, 2015, 165. doi:10.2147/vhrm.s70907.

[24] Ng, Chi-Fai, Chui-Ping Lee, Allen L. Ho, and Vivian W.y. Lee. "Effect of Niacin on Erectile Function in Men Suffering Erectile Dysfunction and Dyslipidemia." *The Journal of Sexual Medicine* 8, no. 10 (2011): 2883-893. doi:10.1111/j.1743-6109.2011.02414.x.

[25] Ooi, Esther M., Gerald F. Watts, Dick C. Chan, Jing Pang, Vijay S. Tenneti, Sandra J. Hamilton, Sally P. Mccormick, Santica M. Marcovina, and P. Hugh R. Barrett. "Effects of Extended-Release Niacin on the Postprandial Metabolism of Lp(a) and ApoB-100–Containing Lipoproteins in Statin-Treated Men With Type 2 Diabetes MellitusSignificance." *Arterioscler Thromb Vasc Biol Arteriosclerosis, Thrombosis, and Vascular Biology* 35, no. 12 (2015): 2686-693. doi:10.1161/atvbaha.115.306136.

[26] Premkumar, Vummidi Giridhar, Srinivasan Yuvaraj, Sivaprakasam Sathish, Palanivel Shanthi, and Panchanatham Sachdanandam. "Anti-angiogenic Potential of CoenzymeQ10, Riboflavin and Niacin in Breast Cancer Patients Undergoing Tamoxifen Therapy." *Vascular Pharmacology* 48, no. 4-6 (2008): 191-201. doi:10.1016/j.vph.2008.02.003.

[27] Moriarty, Patrick M., James Backes, Julie-Ann Dutton, Jianghua He, Janelle F. Ruisinger, and Kristin Schmelzle. "Apple Pectin for the Reduction of Niacin-induced Flushing." *Journal of Clinical Lipidology* 7, no. 2 (2013): 140-46. doi:10.1016/j.jacl.2012.11.005.

[28] Savinova, Olga V., Kristi Fillaus, William S. Harris, and Gregory C. Shearer. "Effects of Niacin and Omega-3 Fatty Acids on the Apolipoproteins in Overweight Patients with Elevated Triglycerides and Reduced HDL Cholesterol." *Atherosclerosis* 240, no. 2 (2015): 520-25. doi:10.1016/j.atherosclerosis.2015.04.793.

[29] Rao, Madhumathi, Michael Steffes, Andrew Bostom, and Joachim H. Ix. "Effect of Niacin on FGF23 Concentration in Chronic Kidney Disease." *American Journal of Nephrology Am J Nephrol* 39, no. 6 (2014): 484-90. doi:10.1159/000362424.

[30] Yasmeen, G. et al. "Association of High-density Lipoprotein Cholesterol with Improvement of Endothelial Dysfunction Recovery in Renovascular Disease." *Iran J Kidney Dis.* 9, no. 1 (January 2015): 39-45.

[31] "Effects of Extended-Release Niacin with Laropiprant in High-Risk Patients." *New England Journal of Medicine N Engl J Med* 371, no. 3 (2014): 203-12. doi:10.1056/nejmoa1300955.

[32] Poly C, Massaro JM, Seshadri S, Wolf PA, Cho E, Krall E, Jacques PF, Au R. The relation of dietary choline to cognitive performance and white-matter hyperintensity in the Framingham Offspring Cohort. Am J Clin Nutr. 2011 Dec;94(6):1584-91. doi: 10.3945/ajcn.110.008938. Epub 2011 Nov 9.

[33] Lu MS, Fang YJ, Pan ZZ, Zhong X, Zheng MC, Chen YM, Zhang CX. Choline and betaine intake and colorectal cancer risk in Chinese population: a case-control study. PLoS One. 2015 Mar 18;10(3):e0118661. doi: 10.1371/journal.pone.0118661. eCollection 2015.

[34] Blusztajn JK, Mellott TJ. Choline nutrition programs brain development via DNA and histone methylation. Cent Nerv Syst Agents Med Chem. 2012 Jun;12(2):82-94.

[35] Bjelland I, Tell GS, Vollset SE, Konstantinova S, Ueland PM. Choline in anxiety and depression: the Hordaland Health Study. Am J Clin Nutr. 2009 Oct;90(4):1056-60. doi: 10.3945/ajcn.2009.27493. Epub 2009 Aug 5.

[36] Rajaie S, Esmaillzadeh A. Dietary choline and betaine intakes and risk of cardiovascular diseases: review of epidemiological evidence. ARYA Atheroscler. 2011 Summer;7(2):78-86.

[37] Jaiswal SK, Sukla KK, et al. Choline metabolic pathway gene polymorphisms and risk for Down syndrome: An association study in a population with folate-homocysteine metabolic impairment. Eur J Clin Nutr. 2017 Jan;71(1):45-50. doi: 10.1038/ejcn.2016.190. Epub 2016 Sep 28.

[38] Kumar, Malavika Vinod, and S. Rajagopalan. "Trial Using Multiple Micronutrient Food Supplement and Its Effect on Cognition." *Indian J Pediatr The Indian Journal of Pediatrics* 75, no. 7 (2008): 671-78. doi:10.1007/s12098-008-0127-1.

[39] Neiva, Rodrigo F., Khalaf Al-Shammari, Francisco H. Nociti, Stephen Soehren, and Hom-Lay Wang. "Effects of Vitamin-B Complex Supplementation on Periodontal Wound Healing." *Journal of Periodontology* 76, no. 7 (2005): 1084-091. doi:10.1902/jop.2005.76.7.1084.

[40] Celebi, S. et al. "Efficacy of Dexpanthenol for Pediatric Post-tonsillectomy Pain and Wound Healing." *Ann Otol Rhinol Laryngol* 122, no. 7 (July 2013): 464-67.

[41] Udompataikul, M., and W. Srisatwaja. "Comparative Trial of Moisturizer Containing Licochalcone A vs. Hydrocortisone Lotion in the Treatment of Childhood Atopic Dermatitis: A Pilot Study." *Journal of the European Academy of Dermatology and Venereology* 25, no. 6 (2010): 660-65. doi:10.1111/j.1468-3083.2010.03845.x.

[42] Camargo, FB. et al. "Skin Moisturizing Effects of Panthenol-based Formulations." *J Cosmet Sci.* 62, no. 4 (July/August 2011): 361-70.

[43] Wolff, Helmut H., and Meinhard Kieser. "Hamamelis in Children with Skin Disorders and Skin Injuries: Results of an Observational Study." *European Journal of Pediatrics Eur J Pediatr* 166, no. 9 (2006): 943-48. doi:10.1007/s00431-006-0363-1.

[44] Evans, Malkanthi, John Rumberger, Isao Azumano, Joseph Napolitano, Danielle Citrolo, and Toshikazu Kamiya. "Pantethine, a Derivative of Vitamin

B5, Favorably Alters Total, LDL and Non-HDL Cholesterol in Low to Moderate Cardiovascular Risk Subjects Eligible for Statin Therapy: A Triple-blinded Placebo and Diet-controlled Investigation." *VHRM Vascular Health and Risk Management*, 2014, 89. doi:10.2147/vhrm.s57116.

[45] Poverennova, IE. et al. "Efficacy and Tolerability of Pantogam Activ in Patients with Partial Epilepsy." *Zh Nevrol Psikhiatr Im S S Korsakova* 111, no. 2 (2011): 54-59.

[46] Toromanyan, Edward, Gayane Aslanyan, Elmira Amroyan, Emil Gabrielyan, and Alexander Panossian. "Efficacy of Slim339® in Reducing Body Weight of Overweight and Obese Human Subjects." *Phytother. Res. Phytotherapy Research* 21, no. 12 (2007): 1177-181. doi:10.1002/ptr.2231.

[47] Hayflick, Susan J. "Defective Pantothenate Metabolism and Neurodegeneration." *Biochm. Soc. Trans. Biochemical Society Transactions* 42, no. 4 (2014): 1063-068. doi:10.1042/bst20140098.

[48] Babaei, AH. "A Randomized Comparison of Vitamin B6 and Dimenhydrinate in the Treatment of Nausea and Vomiting in Early Pregnancy." *Iran J Nurs Midwifery Res.* 19, no. 2 (March 2014): 199-202.

[49] Masoumi, Seyedeh Zahra, Maryam Ataollahi, and Khodayar Oshvandi. "Effect of Combined Use of Calcium and Vitamin B6 on Premenstrual Syndrome Symptoms: A Randomized Clinical Trial." *Journal of Caring Sciences J Caring Sci* 5, no. 1 (2016): 67-73. doi:10.15171/jcs.2016.007.

[50] Xue, J. "Clinical Characteristics and Prognosis Analysis of Vitamin B6 Responsive Infantile Spasms." *Zhonghua Er Ke Za Zhi* 54, no. 2 (February 2016): 141-44.

[51] Hinz, Marty, Alvin Stein, Ted Cole, Beth Mcdougall, and Mark Westaway. "Parkinson's Disease Managing Reversible Neurodegeneration." *NDT Neuropsychiatric Disease and Treatment*, 2016, 763. doi:10.2147/ndt.s98367.

[52] Bessler, H. "Vitamin B6 Modifies the Immune Cross-Talk between Mononuclear and Colon Carcinoma Cells." *Folia Biol (Praha).* 62, no. 1 (2016): 47-52.

[53] Aufiero, Elaine, Todd P. Stitik, Patrick M. Foye, and Boqing Chen. "Pyridoxine Hydrochloride Treatment of Carpal Tunnel Syndrome: A Review." *Nutrition Reviews* 62, no. 3 (2004): 96-104. doi:10.1111/j.1753-4887.2004.tb00030.x.

[54] Almeida, O. P., A. H. Ford, V. Hirani, V. Singh, F. M. Vanbockxmeer, K. Mccaul, and L. Flicker. "B Vitamins to Enhance Treatment Response to Antidepressants in Middle-aged and Older Adults: Results from the B-VITAGE Randomised, Double-blind, Placebo-controlled Trial." *The British Journal of Psychiatry* 205, no. 6 (2014): 450-57. doi:10.1192/bjp.bp.114.145177.

[55] Douaud, Gwenaëlle, Helga Refsum, Celeste A. De Jager, Robin Jacoby, Thomas E. Nichols, Stephen M. Smith, and A. David Smith. "Preventing Alzheimer's Disease-related Gray Matter Atrophy by B-vitamin Treatment." *Proceedings of the National Academy of Sciences Proc Natl Acad Sci USA* 110, no. 23 (2013): 9523-528. doi:10.1073/pnas.1301816110.

[56] Gariballa, Salah E., Sarah J. Forster, and Hilary J. Powers. "Effects of Mixed Dietary Supplements on Total Plasma Homocysteine Concentrations (tHcy): A Randomized, Double-Blind, Placebo-Controlled Trial." *International Journal for Vitamin and Nutrition Research* 82, no. 4 (2012): 260-66. doi:10.1024/0300-9831/a000118.

[57] Chalermchai, T., K. Tantiphlachiva, H. Suwanrusme, N. Voravud, and V. Sriuranpong. "Randomized Trial of Two Different Doses of Pyridoxine in the Prevention of Capecitabine-associated Palmar-plantar Erythrodysesthesia." *Asia-Pacific Journal of Clinical Oncology* 6, no. 3 (2010): 155-60. doi:10.1111/j.1743-7563.2010.01311.x.

[58] Sedel, Frédéric, Caroline Papeix, Agnès Bellanger, Valérie Touitou, Christine Lebrun-Frenay, Damien Galanaud, Olivier Gout, Olivier Lyon-Caen, and Ayman Tourbah. High Doses of Biotin in Chronic Progressive Multiple Sclerosis: A Pilot Study. *Multiple Sclerosis and Related Disorders* 4, no. 2 (2015): 159-69. doi:10.1016/j.msard.2015.01.005.

[59] Ogawa, Y. et al. Prospective Study of Biotin Treatment in Patients with Erythema Due to Gefitinib or Erlotinib. *Gan To Kagaku Ryoho.* 41, no. 4 (April 2014): 517-22.

[60] Oguma, Shiro, Itiro Ando, Takuo Hirose, Kazuhito Totsune, Hiroshi Sekino, Hiroshi Sato, Yutaka Imai, and Masako Fujiwara. Biotin Ameliorates Muscle Cramps of Hemodialysis Patients: A Prospective Trial. *Tohoku J. Exp. Med. The Tohoku Journal of Experimental Medicine* 227, no. 3 (2012): 217-23. doi:10.1620/tjem.227.217.

[61] Albarracin, Cesar, Burcham Fuqua, Jeff Geohas, Vijaya Juturu, Manley R. Finch, and James R. Komorowski. Combination of Chromium and Biotin Improves Coronary Risk Factors in Hypercholesterolemic Type 2 Diabetes Mellitus: A Placebo-Controlled, Double-Blind Randomized Clinical Trial.

*Journal of the CardioMetabolic Syndrome J CardioMetab Syndrome* 2, no. 2 (2007): 91-97. doi:10.1111/j.1559-4564.2007.06366.x.

62 Singer, Gregory M., and Jeff Geohas. The Effect of Chromium Picolinate and Biotin Supplementation on Glycemic Control in Poorly Controlled Patients with Type 2 Diabetes Mellitus: A Placebo-Controlled, Double-Blinded, Randomized Trial. *Diabetes Technology & Therapeutics* 8, no. 6 (2006): 636-43. doi:10.1089/dia.2006.8.636.

63 Venkataraman, Viswanathan, Debasis Panigrahi, Padma Balaji, and Rafat Jamal. Biotinidase Deficiency in Childhood. *Neurol India Neurology India* 61, no. 4 (2013): 411. doi:10.4103/0028-3886.117614.

64 Boccaletti, V., E. Zendri, G. Giordano, L. Gnetti, and G. De Panfilis. Familial Uncombable Hair Syndrome: Ultrastructural Hair Study and Response to Biotin. *Pediatric Dermatology Pediatr Dermatol* 24, no. 3 (2007). doi:10.1111/j.1525-1470.2007.00385.x.

65 Khalidi, N., Wesley, J. Thoene, Whitehouse Wm, and W. Baker. Biotin Deficiency in a Patient with Short Bowel Syndrome during Home Parenteral Nutrition. *Journal of Parenteral and Enteral Nutrition* 8, no. 3 (1984): 311-14. doi:10.1177/0148607184008003311.

66 Hochman, LG. et al. Brittle Nails: Response to Daily Biotin Supplementation. *Cutis* 51, no. 4 (April 1993): 303-05.

67 Dabbagh, O., J. Brismar, G.g. Gascon, and P.t. Ozand. The Clinical Spectrum of Biotin-treatable Encephalopathies in Saudi Arabia. *Brain and Development* 16 (1994): 72-80. doi:10.1016/0387-7604(94)90099-x.

68 Wozniak, Janet, Stephen V. Faraone, James Chan, Laura Tarko, Mariely Hernandez, Jacqueline Davis, K. Yvonne Woodworth, and Joseph Biederman. "A Randomized Clinical Trial of High Eicosapentaenoic Acid Omega-3 Fatty Acids and Inositol as Monotherapy and in Combination in the Treatment of Pediatric Bipolar Spectrum Disorders." *J. Clin. Psychiatry The Journal of Clinical Psychiatry*, 2015, 1548-555. doi:10.4088/jcp.14m09267.

69 D'anna, Rosario, Antonino Di Benedetto, Angela Scilipoti, Angelo Santamaria, Maria Lieta Interdonato, Elisabetta Petrella, Isabella Neri, Basilio Pintaudi, Francesco Corrado, and Fabio Facchinetti. "Myo-inositol Supplementation for Prevention of Gestational Diabetes in Obese Pregnant Women." *Obstetrics & Gynecology* 126, no. 2 (2015): 310-15. doi:10.1097/aog.0000000000000958.

[70] Calogero, A. E., G. Gullo, S. La Vignera, R. A. Condorelli, and A. Vaiarelli. "Myoinositol Improves Sperm Parameters and Serum Reproductive Hormones in Patients with Idiopathic Infertility: A Prospective Double-blind Randomized Placebo-controlled Study." *Andrology* 3, no. 3 (2015): 491-95. doi:10.1111/andr.12025.

[71] Kamenov, Zdravko, Georgi Kolarov, Antoaneta Gateva, Gianfranco Carlomagno, and Alessandro D. Genazzani. "Ovulation Induction with Myo-inositol Alone and in Combination with Clomiphene Citrate in Polycystic Ovarian Syndrome Patients with Insulin Resistance." *Gynecological Endocrinology* 31, no. 2 (2014): 131-35. doi:10.3109/09513590.2014.964640.

[72] Brusco, GF. Et al "Inositol: Effects on Oocyte Quality in Patients Undergoing ICSI. An Open Study." *Eur Rev Med Pharmacol Sci.* 14, no. 6 (June 2010): 555-61.

[73] Rizzo, P. et al "Effect of the Treatment with Myo-inositol plus Folic Acid plus Melatonin in Comparison with a Treatment with Myo-inositol plus Folic Acid on Oocyte Quality and Pregnancy Outcome in IVF Cycles. A Prospective, Clinical Trial." *Eur Rev Med Pharmacol Sci.* 14, no. 6 (June 2010): 555-61.

[74] Carey, P. D., J. Warwick, B. H. Harvey, D. J. Stein, and S. Seedat. "Single Photon Emission Computed Tomography (SPECT) in Obsessive–Compulsive Disorder Before and After Treatment with Inositol." *Metabolic Brain Disease Metab Brain Dis* 19, no. 1/2 (2004): 125-34. doi:10.1023/b:mebr.0000027423.34733.12.

[75] Palatnik, Alex, Katerina Frolov, Mendel Fux, and Jonathan Benjamin. "Double-Blind, Controlled, Crossover Trial of Inositol Versus Fluvoxamine for the Treatment of Panic Disorder." *Journal of Clinical Psychopharmacology* 21, no. 3 (2001): 335-39. doi:10.1097/00004714-200106000-00014.

[76] Carlomagno, Gianfranco, Vittorio Unfer, Silvia Buffo, and Francesco D'ambrosio. "Myo-inositol in the Treatment of Premenstrual Dysphoric Disorder." *Human Psychopharmacology: Clinical and Experimental Hum. Psychopharmacol Clin Exp* 26, no. 7 (2011): 526-30. doi:10.1002/hup.1241.

[77] Boonyarangkul A, Vinayanuvattikhun N, Chiamchanya C, Visutakul P. Comparative Study of the Effects of Tamoxifen Citrate and Folate on Semen Quality of the Infertile Male with Semen Abnormality. J Med Assoc Thai. 2015 Nov;98(11):1057-63.

[78] Cheong M, Xiao HY, Tay V, Karakochuk CD, Liu YA, Harvey S, Lamers Y, Houghton LA, Kitts DD, Green TJ. Folic acid fortified milk increases blood folate to concentrations associated with a very low risk of neural tube defects in Singaporean women of childbearing age. Asia Pac J Clin Nutr. 2016;25(1):62-70. doi: 10.6133/apjcn.2016.25.1.08.

[79] Huo Y, Li J,et al; CSPPT Investigators. Efficacy of folic acid therapy in primary prevention of stroke among adults with hypertension in China: the CSPPT randomized clinical trial. JAMA. 2015 Apr 7;313(13):1325-35. doi: 10.1001/jama.2015.2274.

[80] Wang L, Li H, Zhou Y, Jin L, Liu J. Low-dose B vitamins supplementation ameliorates cardiovascular risk: a double-blind randomized controlled trial in healthy Chinese elderly. Eur J Nutr. 2015 Apr;54(3):455-64. doi: 10.1007/s00394-014-0729-5. Epub 2014 Jun 11.

[81] Schmoll HJ, Tabernero J, Maroun J, de Braud F, Price T, Van Cutsem E, Hill M, Hoersch S, Rittweger K, Haller DG. Capecitabine Plus Oxaliplatin Compared With Fluorouracil/Folinic Acid As Adjuvant Therapy for Stage III ColonCancer: Final Results of the NO16968 Randomized Controlled Phase III Trial. J Clin Oncol. 2015 Nov 10;33(32):3733-40. doi: 10.1200/JCO.2015.60.9107. Epub 2015 Aug 31.

[82] de Jager CA1, Oulhaj A, Jacoby R, Refsum H, Smith AD. Cognitive and clinical outcomes of homocysteine-lowering B-vitamin treatment in mild cognitive impairment: a randomized controlled trial. Int J Geriatr Psychiatry. 2012 Jun;27(6):592-600. doi: 10.1002/gps.2758. Epub 2011 Jul 21.

[83] Gopinath B, Flood VM, Rochtchina E, Wang JJ, Mitchell P. Homocysteine, folate, vitamin B-12, and 10-y incidence of age-related macular degeneration. Am J Clin Nutr. 2013 Jul;98(1):129-35. doi: 10.3945/ajcn.112.057091. Epub 2013 May 1.

[84] Catena A, Muñoz-Machicao JA, Torres-Espínola FJ, Martínez-Zaldívar C, Diaz-Piedra C, Gil A, Haile G, Györei E, Molloy AM, Decsi T, Koletzko B,Campoy C. Folate and long-chain polyunsaturated fatty acid supplementation during pregnancy has long-term effects on the attention system of 8.5-y-old offspring: a randomized controlled trial. Am J Clin Nutr. 2016 Jan;103(1):115-27. doi: 10.3945/ajcn.115.109108. Epub 2015 Nov 11.

[85] Almeida OP, Ford AH, Hirani V, Singh V, vanBockxmeer FM, McCaul K, Flicker L. B vitamins to enhance treatment response to antidepressants in middle-aged and older adults: results from the B-VITAGE randomised,

double-blind, placebo-controlled trial. Br J Psychiatry. 2014 Dec;205(6):450-7. doi: 10.1192/bjp.bp.114.145177. Epub 2014 Sep 25.

[86] Ko Be, T., A. V. Witte, A. Schnelle, U. Grittner, V. A. Tesky, J. Pantel, J. P. Schuchardt, A. Hahn, J. Bohlken, D. Rujescu, and A. Flo El. "Vitamin B-12 Concentration, Memory Performance, and Hippocampal Structure in Patients with Mild Cognitive Impairment." *American Journal of Clinical Nutrition* 103, no. 4 (2016): 1045-054. doi:10.3945/ajcn.115.116970.

[87] Spence, J. David. "Metabolic Vitamin B12 Deficiency: A Missed Opportunity to Prevent Dementia and Stroke." *Nutrition Research* 36, no. 2 (2016): 109-16. doi:10.1016/j.nutres.2015.10.003.

[88] Zittan, E., M. Preis, I. Asmir, A. Cassel, N. Lindenfeld, S. Alroy, D. A. Halon, B. S. Lewis, A. Shiran, J. E. Schliamser, and M. Y. Flugelman. "High Frequency of Vitamin B12 Deficiency in Asymptomatic Individuals Homozygous to MTHFR C677T Mutation Is Associated with Endothelial Dysfunction and Homocysteinemia." *AJP: Heart and Circulatory Physiology* 293, no. 1 (2007). doi:10.1152/ajpheart.01189.2006.

[89] Goodman. "Vitamin B12 Deficiency. Important New Concepts in Recognition." *Postgrad Med.* 88, no. 3 (September 1, 1990): 147-50.

[90] Goodman. "Vitamin B12 Deficiency. Important New Concepts in Recognition." *Postgrad Med.* 88, no. 3 (September 1, 1990): 147-50.

[91] Goodman. "Vitamin B12 Deficiency. Important New Concepts in Recognition." *Postgrad Med.* 88, no. 3 (September 1, 1990): 147-50.

[92] Goodman. "Vitamin B12 Deficiency. Important New Concepts in Recognition." *Postgrad Med.* 88, no. 3 (September 1, 1990): 147-50.

[93] Chapman, L.e., A.l. Darling, and J.e. Brown. "Association between Metformin and Vitamin B12 Deficiency in Patients with Type 2 Diabetes: A Systematic Review and Meta-analysis." *Diabetes & Metabolism*, 2016. doi:10.1016/j.diabet.2016.03.008.

[94] RM, Nemes. "ANEMIA IN INFLAMMATORY BOWEL DISEASE MORE THAN AN EXTRAINTESTINAL COMPLICATION." *Rev Med Chir Soc Med Nat Iasi* 120, no. 1 (Spring 2016): 34-39.

[95] Regland, Björn, Sara Forsmark, Lena Halaouate, Michael Matousek, Birgitta Peilot, Olof Zachrisson, and Carl-Gerhard Gottfries. "Response to Vitamin

B12 and Folic Acid in Myalgic Encephalomyelitis and Fibromyalgia." *PLOS ONE PLoS ONE* 10, no. 4 (2015). doi:10.1371/journal.pone.0124648.

[96] Guo M, Li Y, Li J. Effect of growth hormone, glutamine, and enteral nutrition on intestinal adaptation in patients with short bowel syndrome. Turk J Gastroenterol. 2013;24(6):463-8.

[97] Lima AA, Anstead GM, et al. Effects of glutamine alone or in combination with zinc and vitamin A on growth, intestinal barrier function, stress and satiety-related hormones in Brazilian shantytown children. Clinics (Sao Paulo). 2014;69(4):225-33.

[98] Huang JS, Wu CL, Fan CW, Chen WH, Yeh KY, Chang PH. Intravenous glutamine appears to reduce the severity of symptomatic platinum-induced neuropathy: a prospective randomized study. J Chemother. 2015 Aug;27(4):235-40. doi: 10.1179/1973947815Y.0000000011. Epub 2015 Mar 23.

[99] Song QH, Xu RM, Zhang QH, Shen GQ, Ma M, Zhao XP, Guo YH, Wang Y. Glutamine supplementation and immune function during heavy load training. Int J Clin Pharmacol Ther. 2015 May;53(5):372-6. doi: 10.5414/CP202227.

[100] Mansour A, Mohajeri-Tehrani MR, et al. Effect of glutamine supplementation on cardiovascular risk factors in patients with type 2 diabetes. Nutrition. 2015 Jan;31(1):119-26. doi: 10.1016/j.nut.2014.05.014. Epub 2014 Jun 23.

[101] Tsujimoto T, Yamamoto L, Wasa M, Takenaka Y, Nakahara S, Takagi T, Tsugane M, Hayashi N, Maeda K, Inohara H2, Uejima E, Ito T. L-glutamine decreases the severity of mucositis induced by chemoradiotherapy in patients with locally advanced head and neck cancer: a double-blind, randomized, placebo-controlled trial. Oncol Rep. 2015 Jan;33(1):33-9. doi: 10.3892/or.2014.3564. Epub 2014 Oct 23.

[102] Laviano A, Molfino A, Lacaria MT, Canelli A, De Leo S, Preziosa I, Rossi Fanelli F. Glutamine supplementation favors weight loss in nondieting obese female patients. A pilot study. Eur J Clin Nutr. 2014 Nov;68(11):1264-6. doi: 10.1038/ejcn.2014.184. Epub 2014 Sep 17.

[103] Nishizaki K, Ikegami H, Tanaka Y, Imai R, Matsumura H. Effects of supplementation with a combination of β-hydroxy-β-methyl butyrate, L-arginine, and L-glutamine on postoperative recovery of quadriceps muscle

strength after total knee arthroplasty. Asia Pac J Clin Nutr. 2015;24(3):412-20. doi: 10.6133/apjcn.2015.24.3.01.

[104] Kuhn KS, Muscaritoli M, Wischmeyer P, Stehle P. Glutamine as indispensable nutrient in oncology: experimental and clinical evidence. Eur J Nutr. 2010 Jun;49(4):197-210. doi: 10.1007/s00394-009-0082-2. Epub 2009 Nov 21.

[105] Mauras N, Xing D, Fox LA, Englert K, Darmaun D. Effects of glutamine on glycemic control during and after exercise in adolescents with type 1 diabetes: a pilot study. Diabetes Care. 2010 Sep;33(9):1951-3. doi: 10.2337/dc10-0275. Epub 2010 Jun 28.

[106] Salvadore G, van der Veen JW, et al. An investigation of amino-acid neurotransmitters as potential predictors of clinical improvement to ketamine in depression. Int J Neuropsychopharmacol. 2012 Sep;15(8):1063-72. doi: 10.1017/S1461145711001593. Epub 2011 Nov 1.

[107] Kohda D. Structural Basis of Protein Asn-Glycosylation by Oligosaccharyltransferases. Adv Exp Med Biol. 2018;1104:171-199. doi: 10.1007/978-981-13-2158-0_9.

[108] No authors listed. Urea Cycle: Steps Involved and Metabolic Disorders | Protein Metabolism found at http://www.biologydiscussion.com/proteins/metabolism-proteins/urea-cycle-steps-involved-and-metabolic-disorders-protein-metabolism/17201. Accessed 12/29/18.

[109] Marquezi ML, Roschel HA, dos Santa Costa A, Sawada LA, Lancha AH Jr. Effect of aspartate and asparagine supplementation on fatigue determinants in intense exercise. Int J Sport Nutr Exerc Metab. 2003 Mar;13(1):65-75.

[110] No authors listed. Urea Cycle: Steps Involved and Metabolic Disorders | Protein Metabolism found at http://www.biologydiscussion.com/proteins/metabolism-proteins/urea-cycle-steps-involved-and-metabolic-disorders-protein-metabolism/17201. Accessed 12/29/18.

[111] Minshawi NF, Wink LK, et al. A randomized, placebo-controlled trial of D-cycloserine for the enhancement of social skills training in autism spectrum disorders. Mol Autism. 2016 Jan 14;7:2. doi: 10.1186/s13229-015-0062-8. eCollection 2016.

112 Levinson CA, Rodebaugh TL, Fewell L, Kass AE, Riley EN, Stark L, McCallum K, Lenze EJ. D-Cycloserine facilitation of exposure therapy improves weight regain in patients with anorexia nervosa: a pilot randomized controlled trial. J Clin Psychiatry. 2015 Jun;76(6):e787-93. doi: 10.4088/JCP.14m09299.

113 de Kleine RA, Smits JA, Hendriks GJ, Becker ES, van Minnen A. Extinction learning as a moderator of d-cycloserine efficacy for enhancing exposure therapy in posttraumatic stress disorder. J Anxiety Disord. 2015 Aug;34:63-7. doi: 10.1016/j.janxdis.2015.06.005. Epub 2015 Jun 14.

114 Wilhelm S, Buhlmann U, Tolin DF, Meunier SA, Pearlson GD, Reese HE, Cannistraro P, Jenike MA, Rauch SL. Augmentation of behavior therapy with D-cycloserine for obsessive-compulsive disorder. Am J Psychiatry. 2008 Mar;165(3):335-41; quiz 409. doi: 10.1176/appi.ajp.2007.07050776. Epub 2008 Feb 1.

115 Heresco-Levy U, Gelfin G, Bloch B, Levin R, Edelman S, Javitt DC, Kremer I. A randomized add-on trial of high-dose D-cycloserine for treatment-resistant depression. Int J Neuropsychopharmacol. 2013 Apr;16(3):501-6. doi: 10.1017/S1461145712000910. Epub 2012 Sep 17.

116 Forsyth JK, Bachman P, Mathalon DH, Roach BJ, Asarnow RF. Augmenting NMDA receptor signaling boosts experience-dependent neuroplasticity in the adult human brain. Proc Natl Acad Sci U S A. 2015 Dec 15;112(50):15331-6. doi: 10.1073/pnas.1509262112. Epub 2015 Nov 30.

117 Cain CK, McCue M, Bello I, Creedon T, Tang DI, Laska E, Goff DC. d-Cycloserine augmentation of cognitive remediation in schizophrenia. Schizophr Res. 2014 Mar;153(1-3):177-83. doi: 10.1016/j.schres.2014.01.016. Epub 2014 Jan 30.

118 Kiefer F, Kirsch M, et al. Effects of D-cycloserine on extinction of mesolimbic cue reactivity in alcoholism: a randomized placebo-controlled trial. Psychopharmacology (Berl). 2015 Jul;232(13):2353-62. doi: 10.1007/s00213-015-3882-5. Epub 2015 Feb 21.

119 Tyan ML. Effects of inositol, LiCl, and heparin on the antibody responses to SRBC by normal and immunodeficient XID mice. Proc Soc Exp Biol Med. 2000 Jul;224(3):187-90.

[120] Leombruni P, Miniotti M, et al. A randomised controlled trial comparing duloxetine and acetyl L-carnitine in fibromyalgic patients: preliminary data. Clin Exp Rheumatol. 2015 Jan-Feb;33(1 Suppl 88):S82-5. Epub 2015 Mar 18.

[121] Lee BJ, Lin JS, Lin YC, Lin PT. Antiinflammatory effects of L-carnitine supplementation (1000 mg/d) in coronary artery disease patients. Nutrition. 2015 Mar;31(3):475-9. doi: 10.1016/j.nut.2014.10.001. Epub 2014 Oct 16.

[122] Remington R, Bechtel C, et al. A Phase II Randomized Clinical Trial of a Nutritional Formulation for Cognition and Mood in Alzheimer's Disease. J Alzheimers Dis. 2015;45(2):395-405. doi: 10.3233/JAD-142499.

[123] L-Carnitine-supplementation in advanced pancreatic cancer (CARPAN)--a randomized multicentre trial.
Kraft M, Kraft K, Gärtner S, Mayerle J, Simon P, Weber E, Schütte K, Stieler J, Koula-Jenik H, Holzhauer P, Gröber U, Engel G, Müller C, Feng YS, Aghdassi A, Nitsche C, Malfertheiner P, Patrzyk M, Kohlmann T, Lerch MM. Nutr J. 2012 Jul 23;11:52. doi: 10.1186/1475-2891-11-52.

[124] Oncologist. 2013;18(11):1190-1. doi: 10.1634/theoncologist.2013-0061. Epub 2013 Oct 8.
Campone M1, Berton-Rigaud D, Joly-Lobbedez F, Baurain JF, Rolland F, Stenzl A, Fabbro M, van Dijk M, Pinkert J, Schmelter T, de Bont N, Pautier P. A double-blind, randomized phase II study to evaluate the safety and efficacy of acetyl-L-carnitine in the prevention of sagopilone-induced peripheral neuropathy.

[125] Leombruni P, Miniotti M, et al. A randomised controlled trial comparing duloxetine and acetyl L-carnitine in fibromyalgic patients: preliminary data. Clin Exp Rheumatol. 2015 Jan-Feb;33(1 Suppl 88):S82-5. Epub 2015 Mar 18.

[126] Salas-Huetos A, Rosique-Esteban N, et al. The Effect of Nutrients and Dietary Supplements on Sperm Quality Parameters: A Systematic Review and Meta-Analysis of Randomized Clinical Trials. Adv Nutr. 2018 Nov 1;9(6):833-848. doi: 10.1093/advances/nmy057.

[127] Stephens FB, Wall BT, Marimuthu K, Shannon CE, Constantin-Teodosiu D, Macdonald IA, Greenhaff PL. Skeletal muscle carnitine loading increases energy expenditure, modulates fuel metabolism gene networks and prevents body fat accumulation in humans. J Physiol. 2013 Sep 15;591(18):4655-66. doi: 10.1113/jphysiol.2013.255364. Epub 2013 Jul 1.

128 Sawicka AK, Hartmane D, et al. l-Carnitine Supplementation in Older Women. A Pilot Study on Aging Skeletal Muscle Mass and Function. Nutrients. 2018 Feb 23;10(2). pii: E255. doi: 10.3390/nu10020255.

129 Zhang W, Li P, et al. [Safety and efficacy of L-carnitine and tadalafil for late-onset hypogonadism with ED: a randomized controlled multicenter clinical trial]. Zhonghua Nan Ke Xue. 2014 Feb;20(2):133-7.
[Article in Chinese]

130 Jones PJ, Senanayake VK, et al. DHA-enriched high-oleic acid canola oil improves lipid profile and lowers predicted cardiovascular disease risk in the canola oil multicenter randomized controlled trial. Am J Clin Nutr. 2014 Jul;100(1):88-97. doi: 10.3945/ajcn.113.081133. Epub 2014 May 14.

131 Bellenghi M, Puglisi R, et al. SCD5-induced oleic acid production reduces melanoma malignancy by intracellular retention of SPARC and cathepsin B. J Pathol. 2015 Jul;236(3):315-25. doi: 10.1002/path.4535. Epub 2015 Apr 20.

132 Khan AA, Alanazi AM, Jabeen M, Parvez MK, Wahab R, Abdelhameed AS, Chauhan A. Biophysical Interactions of Novel Oleic Acid Conjugate and its Anticancer Potential in HeLa Cells. J Fluoresc. 2015 May;25(3):519-25. doi: 10.1007/s10895-015-1512-6. Epub 2015 Feb 1.

133 Moon HS, Batirel S, Mantzoros CS. Alpha linolenic acid and oleic acid additively down-regulate malignant potential and positively cross-regulate AMPK/S6 axis in OE19 and OE33 esophageal cancer cells. Metabolism. 2014 Nov;63(11):1447-54. doi: 10.1016/j.metabol.2014.07.009. Epub 2014 Jul 25.

134 Moreira Alves RD, Boroni Moreira AP, Macedo VS, Bressan J, de Cássia Gonçalves Alfenas R, Mattes R, Brunoro Costa NM. High-oleic peanuts: new perspective to attenuate glucose homeostasis disruption and inflammation related obesity. Obesity (Silver Spring). 2014 Sep;22(9):1981-8. doi: 10.1002/oby.20825. Epub 2014 Jun 27.

135 Sales-Campos H, Souza PR, Peghini BC, da Silva JS, Cardoso CR. An overview of the modulatory effects of oleic acid in health and disease. Mini Rev Med Chem. 2013 Feb;13(2):201-10

136 Sales-Campos H, Souza PR, Peghini BC, da Silva JS, Cardoso CR. An overview of the modulatory effects of oleic acid in health and disease. Mini Rev Med Chem. 2013 Feb;13(2):201-10

[137] Sales-Campos H, Souza PR, Peghini BC, da Silva JS, Cardoso CR. An overview of the modulatory effects of oleic acid in health and disease. Mini Rev Med Chem. 2013 Feb;13(2):201-10

[138] Hadj Ahmed S, Kharroubi W, et al. Correlation of trans fatty acids with the severity of coronary artery disease lesions. Lipids Health Dis. 2018 Mar 15;17(1):52. doi: 10.1186/s12944-018-0699-3.

[139] Bi, Xinyan, et al. "Prevalence of Vitamin D Deficiency in Singapore: Its Implications to Cardiovascular Risk Factors." *PLOS ONE PLoS ONE* 11, no. 1 (January 22, 2016). doi:10.1371/journal.pone.0147616.

[140] S, Basit, et al. "Vitamin D in Health and Disease: A Literature Review." *Br J Biomed Sci* 70, no. 4 (2013): 161-72.

[141] B. Heidari, et al. "Restorative Effect of Vitamin D Deficiency on Knee Pain and Quadriceps Muscle Strength in Knee Osteoarthritis." *Acta Med Iran* 53, no. 8 (August 2015): 466-70.

[142] Orme, Rowan P., et al. "The Role of Vitamin D3 in the Development and Neuroprotection of Midbrain Dopamine Neurons." *Vitamin D Hormone Vitamins & Hormones*, 2016, 273-97. doi:10.1016/bs.vh.2015.10.007.

[143] Sikoglu, Elif M., et al. "Vitamin D 3 Supplemental Treatment for Mania in Youth with Bipolar Spectrum Disorders." *Journal of Child and Adolescent Psychopharmacology* 25, no. 5 (2015): 415-24. doi:10.1089/cap.2014.0110.

[144] Peng, Wen, et al. "1,25 Dihydroxyvitamin D3 Inhibits the Proliferation of Thyroid Cancer Stem-like Cells via Cell Cycle Arrest." *Endocrine Research* 41, no. 2 (2016): 71-80. doi:10.3109/07435800.2015.1037048.

[145] Nwosu, et al. "The Effects of Vitamin D Supplementation on Hepatic Dysfunction, Vitamin D Status, and Glycemic Control in Children and Adolescents with Vitamin D Deficiency and Either Type 1 or Type 2 Diabetes Mellitus." *PLoS ONE* 9, no. 6 (2014). doi:10.1371/journal.pone.0099646.

[146] The, N. S., et al. "Vitamin D in Youth with Type 1 Diabetes: Prevalence of Insufficiency and Association with Insulin Resistance in the SEARCH Nutrition Ancillary Study." *Diabet. Med. Diabetic Medicine* 30, no. 11 (2013): 1324-332. doi:10.1111/dme.12297.

[147] Jamall, Omer A., et al. "Prevalence and Correlates of Vitamin D Deficiency in Adults after Traumatic Brain Injury." *Clin Endocrinol Clinical Endocrinology*, 2016. doi:10.1111/cen.13045.

[148] Wepner, Florian, et al. "Effects of Vitamin D on Patients with Fibromyalgia Syndrome: A Randomized Placebo-controlled Trial." *Pain* 155, no. 2 (2014): 261-68. doi:10.1016/j.pain.2013.10.002.

[149] Parikh, Coral, et al. "Vitamin D and Clinical Outcomes in Dialysis." *Semin Dial Seminars in Dialysis* 28, no. 6 (2015): 604-09. doi:10.1111/sdi.12446.

[150] Randhawa M, Rossetti D, Leyden JJ, Fantasia J, Zeichner J, Cula GO, Southall M, Tucker-Samaras S. One-year topical stabilized retinol treatment improves photodamaged skin in a double-blind, vehicle-controlled trial. J Drugs Dermatol. 2015 Mar;14(3):271-80.

[151] Randhawa M, Rossetti D, Leyden JJ, Fantasia J, Zeichner J, Cula GO, Southall M, Tucker-Samaras S. One-year topical stabilized retinol treatment improves photodamaged skin in a double-blind, vehicle-controlled trial. J Drugs Dermatol. 2015 Mar;14(3):271-80.
[152] Veraldi S, Barbareschi M, Guanziroli E, Bettoli V, Minghetti S, Capitanio B, Sinagra JL, Sedona P, Schianchi R. Treatment of mild to moderate acne with a fixed combination of hydroxypinacolone retinoate, retinolglycospheres and papain glycospheres. G Ital Dermatol Venereol. 2015 Apr;150(2):143-7.

[153] Ho ET, Trookman NS, Sperber BR, Rizer RL, Spindler R, Sonti S, Gotz V, Mehta R. A randomized, double-blind, controlled comparative trial of the anti-aging properties of non-prescription tri-retinol 1.1% vs. prescription tretinoin 0.025%. J Drugs Dermatol. 2012 Jan;11(1):64-9.

[154] McCauley ME, van den Broek N, Dou L, Othman M. Vitamin A supplementation during pregnancy for maternal and newborn outcomes. Cochrane Database Syst Rev. 2015 Oct 27;(10):CD008666. doi: 10.1002/14651858.CD008666.pub3.

[155] Lucock M, Jones P, et al. Photobiology of vitamins. Nutr Rev. 2018 Jul 1;76(7):512-525. doi: 10.1093/nutrit/nuy013.

[156] McCauley ME, van den Broek N, Dou L, Othman M. Vitamin A supplementation during pregnancy for maternal and newborn outcomes. Cochrane Database Syst Rev. 2015 Oct 27;(10):CD008666. doi: 10.1002/14651858.CD008666.pub3.

[157] Doldo E, Costanza G, et al. Vitamin A, cancer treatment and prevention: the new role of cellular retinol binding proteins. Biomed Res Int. 2015;2015:624627. doi: 10.1155/2015/624627. Epub 2015 Mar 24.

[158] Patel S, Vajdy M. Induction of cellular and molecular immunomodulatory

pathways by vitamin A and flavonoids. Expert Opin Biol Ther. 2015;15(10):1411-28. doi: 10.1517/14712598.2015.1066331. Epub 2015 Jul 17.

[159] Huang Z, Liu Y, et al. Role of Vitamin A in the Immune System. J Clin Med. 2018 Sep 6;7(9). pii: E258. doi: 10.3390/jcm7090258.

[160] Iqbal S, Naseem I. Role of vitamin A in type 2 diabetes mellitus biology: effects of intervention therapy in a deficient state. Nutrition. 2015 Jul-Aug;31(7-8):901-7. doi: 10.1016/j.nut.2014.12.014. Epub 2014 Dec 31.

[161] Ozdemir MA, Yilmaz K, Abdulrezzak U, Muhtaroglu S, Patiroglu T, Karakukcu M, Unal E. The efficacy of vitamin K2 and calcitriol combination on thalassemic osteopathy. J Pediatr Hematol Oncol. 2013 Nov;35(8):623-7. doi: 10.1097/MPH.0000000000000040.

[162] Koitaya N, Sekiguchi M, Tousen Y, Nishide Y, Morita A, Yamauchi J, Gando Y, Miyachi M, Aoki M, Komatsu M, Watanabe F, Morishita K, Ishimi Y. Low-dose vitamin K2 (MK-4) supplementation for 12 months improves bone metabolism and prevents forearm bone loss in postmenopausal Japanese women. J Bone Miner Metab. 2014 Mar;32(2):142-50. doi: 10.1007/s00774-013-0472-7. Epub 2013 May 24.

[163] Knapen MH, Drummen NE, Smit E, Vermeer C, Theuwissen E. Three-year low-dose menaquinone-7 supplementation helps decrease bone loss in healthy postmenopausal women. Osteoporos Int. 2013 Sep;24(9):2499-507. doi: 10.1007/s00198-013-2325-6. Epub 2013 Mar 23.

[164] Forli L, Bollerslev J, Simonsen S, Isaksen GA, Kvamsdal KE, Godang K, Gadeholt G, Pripp AH, Bjortuft O. Dietary vitamin K2 supplement improves bone status after lung and heart transplantation. Transplantation. 2010 Feb 27;89(4):458-64. doi: 10.1097/TP.0b013e3181c46b69.

[165] Kojima K, Tamano M, Akima T, Hashimoto T, Kuniyoshi T, Maeda C, Majima Y, Kusano K, Murohisa T, Iijima M, Hiraishi H. Effect of vitamin K2 on the development of hepatocellular carcinoma in type C cirrhosis. Hepatogastroenterology. 2010 Sep-Oct;57(102-103):1264-7.

[166] Takami A, Asakura H, Nakao S. Menatetrenone, a vitamin K2 analog, ameliorates cytopenia in patients with refractory anemia of myelodysplastic syndrome. Ann Hematol. 2002 Jan;81(1):16-9. Epub 2001 Dec 8.

[167] Knapen MH, Drummen NE, Smit E, Vermeer C, Theuwissen E. Three-year low-dose menaquinone-7 supplementation helps decrease bone loss in

healthy postmenopausal women. Osteoporos Int. 2013 Sep;24(9):2499-507. doi: 10.1007/s00198-013-2325-6. Epub 2013 Mar 23.

168 Bunyaratavej N, Kittimanon N, Jitivirai T, Tongthongthip B. Highly recommended dose of MK4 for osteoporosis. J Med Assoc Thai. 2009 Sep;92 Suppl5:S4-6.

169 ACosentino F, Ceriello A, et al. ddressing cardiovascular risk in type 2 diabetes mellitus: a report from the European Society of Cardiology Cardiovascular Roundtable. Eur Heart J. 2018 Nov 16. doi: 10.1093/eurheartj/ehy677. [Epub ahead of print] No abstract available.

170 Zuchinali P, Souza GC, Aliti G, Botton MR, Goldraich L, Santos KG, Hutz MH, Bandinelli E, Rohde LE. Influence of VKORC1 gene polymorphisms on the effect of oral vitamin K supplementation in over-anticoagulated patients. J Thromb Thrombolysis. 2014 Apr;37(3):338-44. doi: 10.1007/s11239-013-0947-3.

171 Ferland G. Vitamin K and brain function. Semin Thromb Hemost. 2013 Nov;39(8):849-55. doi: 10.1055/s-0033-1357481. Epub 2013 Oct 9.

172 Bristow, Sarah M., Greg D. Gamble, Angela Stewart, Anne M. Horne, and Ian R. Reid. "Acute Effects of Calcium Supplements on Blood Pressure and Blood Coagulation: Secondary Analysis of a Randomised Controlled Trial in Post-menopausal Women." *British Journal of Nutrition Br J Nutr* 114, no. 11 (2015): 1868-874. doi:10.1017/s0007114515003694.

173 Zhao, Yingchun, Rui Cao, Danjun Ma, Hengwei Zhang, Joan Lappe, Robert R. Recker, and Gary Guishan Xiao. "Efficacy of Calcium Supplementation for Human Bone Health by Mass Spectrometry Profiling and Cathepsin K Measurement in Plasma Samples." *J Bone Miner Metab Journal of Bone and Mineral Metabolism* 29, no. 5 (2011): 552-60. doi:10.1007/s00774-010-0251-7.

174 Heaney, R. P., R. R. Recker, P. Watson, and J. M. Lappe. "Phosphate and Carbonate Salts of Calcium Support Robust Bone Building in Osteoporosis." *American Journal of Clinical Nutrition* 92, no. 1 (2010): 101-05. doi:10.3945/ajcn.2009.29085.

175 Rodriguez-Stanley, Sheila, Tanveer Ahmed, Sattar Zubaidi, Susan Riley, Hamid I. Akbarali, Mark H. Mellow, and Philip B. Miner. "Calcium Carbonate Antacids Alter Esophageal Motility in Heartburn Sufferers." *Dig Dis Sci Digestive Diseases and Sciences* 49, no. 11-12 (2004): 1862-867. doi:10.1007/s10620-004-9584-1.

[176] Wang, Yong, Guoqiang Xie, Yuanhang Huang, Han Zhang, Bo Yang, and Zhiguo Mao. "Calcium Acetate or Calcium Carbonate for Hyperphosphatemia of Hemodialysis Patients: A Meta-Analysis." *PLOS ONE PLoS ONE* 10, no. 3 (2015). doi:10.1371/journal.pone.0121376.

[177] Carvalho, Ceci Nunes, Jose Bauer, Patricia Helena Pereira Ferrari, Soraia Fatima Carvalho Souza, Silvio Peixoto Soares, Alessandro Dourado Loguercio, and Antonio Carlos Bombana. "Influence of Calcium Hydroxide Intracanal Medication on Bond Strength of Two Endodontic Resin-based Sealers Assessed by Micropush-out Test." *Dent Traumatol Dental Traumatology* 29, no. 1 (2012): 73-76. doi:10.1111/j.1600-9657.2011.01109.x.

[178] Aykut-Yetkiner, Arzu, Nazan Kara, Mustafa Ateş, Nazan Ersin, and Fahinur Ertuğrul. "Does Casein Phosphopeptid Amorphous Calcium Phosphate Provide Remineralization on White Spot Lesions and Inhibition of Streptococcus Mutans?" *Journal of Clinical Pediatric Dentistry* 38, no. 4 (2014): 302-06. doi:10.17796/jcpd.38.4.b4q401v6m4818215.

[179] Porciani, PF. Et al. "A Clinical Study of the Efficacy of a New Chewing Gum Containing Calcium Hydroxyapatite in Reducing Dentin Hypersensitivity." *J Clin Dent* 25, no. 2 (2014): 32-36.

[180] Reid, Ian R., Ruth Ames, Barbara Mason, Helen E. Reid, Catherine J. Bacon, Mark J. Bolland, Gregory D. Gamble, Andrew Grey, and Anne Horne. "Randomized Controlled Trial of Calcium Supplementation in Healthy, Nonosteoporotic, Older Men." *Arch Intern Med Archives of Internal Medicine* 168, no. 20 (2008): 2276. doi:10.1001/archinte.168.20.2276.

[181] Hammar, M. "Calcium and Magnesium Status in Pregnant Women. A Comparison between Treatment with Calcium and Vitamin C in Pregnant Women with Leg Cramps." *Int J Vitam Nutr Res* 57, no. 2 (1987): 179-83.

[182] Palacios C. The role of nutrients in bone health, from A to Z. Crit Rev Food Sci Nutr. 2006;46(8):621-8.

[183] Landete-Castillejos T, Molina-Quilez I, Estevez JA, Ceacero F, Garcia AJ, Gallego L. Alternative hypothesis for the origin of osteoporosis: the role of Mn. Front Biosci (Elite Ed). 2012 Jan 1;4:1385-90.

[184] Fudalej S, Kołodziejczyk I, Gajda T, Majkowska-Zwolińska B, Wojnar M. Manganese-induced Parkinsonism among ephedrone users and drug policy in Poland. J Addict Med. 2013 Jul-Aug;7(4):302-3. doi: 10.1097/ADM.0b013e3182915dce.

[185] Gaby AR. Natural approaches to epilepsy. Altern Med Rev. 2007 Mar;12(1):9-24.

[186] Li C, Zhou HM. The role of manganese superoxide dismutase in inflammation defense. Enzyme Res. 2011;2011:387176. doi: 10.4061/2011/387176. Epub 2011 Oct 3.

[187] Konzack A, Kietzmann T. Manganese superoxide dismutase in carcinogenesis: friend or foe? Biochem Soc Trans. 2014 Aug;42(4):1012-6. doi: 10.1042/BST20140076.

[188] Chen P, Chakraborty S, et al. Manganese homeostasis in the nervous system. J Neurochem. 2015 Aug;134(4):601-10. doi: 10.1111/jnc.13170. Epub 2015 Jun 16.

[189] Kehl-Fie TE, Skaar EP. Nutritional immunity beyond iron: a role for manganese and zinc. Curr Opin Chem Biol. 2010 Apr;14(2):218-24. doi: 10.1016/j.cbpa.2009.11.008. Epub 2009 Dec 16.

[190] Kehl-Fie TE, Skaar EP. Nutritional immunity beyond iron: a role for manganese and zinc. Curr Opin Chem Biol. 2010 Apr;14(2):218-24. doi: 10.1016/j.cbpa.2009.11.008. Epub 2009 Dec 16.

[191] Penland JG, Johnson PE. Dietary calcium and manganese effects on menstrual cycle symptoms.
Am J Obstet Gynecol. 1993 May;168(5):1417-23.

[192] Zekavat, Omid R., Mohammad Y. Karimi, Aida Amanat, and Farzaneh Alipour. "A Randomised Controlled Trial of Oral Zinc Sulphate for Primary Dysmenorrhoea in Adolescent Females." *Aust N Z J Obstet Gynaecol Australian and New Zealand Journal of Obstetrics and Gynaecology* 55, no. 4 (2015): 369-73. doi:10.1111/ajo.12367.

[193] Nossier, Samia A., Noha E. Naeim, Nawal A. El-Sayed, and Azza A. Abu Zeid. "The Effect of Zinc Supplementation on Pregnancy Outcomes: A Double-blind, Randomised Controlled Trial, Egypt." *British Journal of Nutrition Br J Nutr* 114, no. 02 (2015): 274-85. doi:10.1017/s000711451500166x.

[194] Salari, Soheila, Payam Khomand, Modabber Arasteh, Bahareh Yousefzamani, and Kambiz Hassanzadeh. "Zinc Sulphate: A Reasonable Choice for Depression Management in Patients with Multiple Sclerosis: A Randomized, Double-blind, Placebo-controlled Clinical Trial." *Pharmacological Reports* 67, no. 3 (2015): 606-09. doi:10.1016/j.pharep.2015.01.002.

195 Kurugöl, Zafer, Nuri Bayram, and Tahir Atik. "Effect of Zinc Sulfate on Common Cold in Children: Randomized, Double Blind Study." *Pediatrics International Pediatr Int* 49, no. 6 (2007): 842-47. doi:10.1111/j.1442-200x.2007.02448.x.

196 Chassard, Didier, Roo Kanis, Florence Namour, Eric Evene, Bernard Ntssikoussalabongui, and Valérie Schmitz. "A Single Centre, Open-label, Cross-over Study of Pharmacokinetics Comparing Topical Zinc/clindamycin Gel (Zindaclin®) and Topical Clindamycin Lotion (Dalacin® T) in Subjects with Mild to Moderate Acne." *Journal of Dermatological Treatment* 17, no. 3 (2006): 154-57. doi:10.1080/09546630600727115.

197 Sanchez, J. "Effect of Zinc Amino Acid Chelate and Zinc Sulfate in the Incidence of Respiratory Infection and Diarrhea among Preschool Children in Child Daycare Centers." *Biomedica* 34, no. 1 (January 2014): 79-91. doi:10.1590/S0120-41572014000100011.

198 Khattar, Joe A., Umayya M. Musharrafieh, Hala Tamim, and Ghassan N. Hamadeh. "Topical Zinc Oxide vs. Salicylic Acid?lactic Acid Combination in the Treatment of Warts." *International Journal of Dermatology Int J Dermatol* 46, no. 4 (2007): 427-30. doi:10.1111/j.1365-4632.2006.03138.x.

199 Stebbins, William G., William C. Hanke, and Jeffrey Petersen. "Enhanced Healing of Surgical Wounds of the Lower Leg Using Weekly Zinc Oxide Compression Dressings." *Dermatologic Surgery* 37, no. 2 (2011): 158-65. doi:10.1111/j.1524-4725.2010.01844.x.

200 Kobayashi, Hiroki, Masanori Abe, Kazuyoshi Okada, Ritsukou Tei, Noriaki Maruyama, Fumito Kikuchi, Terumi Higuchi, and Masayoshi Soma. "Oral Zinc Supplementation Reduces the Erythropoietin Responsiveness Index in Patients on Hemodialysis." *Nutrients* 7, no. 5 (2015): 3783-795. doi:10.3390/nu7053783.

201 Smailhodzic, Dzenita, Freekje Van Asten, Anna M. Blom, Frida C. Mohlin, Anneke I. Den Hollander, Johannes P. H. Van De Ven, Ramon A. C. Van Huet, Joannes M. M. Groenewoud, Yuan Tian, Tos T. J. M. Berendschot, Yara T. E. Lechanteur, Sascha Fauser, Chris De Bruijn, Mohamed R. Daha, Gert Jan Van Der Wilt, Carel B. Hoyng, and B. Jeroen Klevering. "Zinc Supplementation Inhibits Complement Activation in Age-Related Macular Degeneration." *PLoS ONE* 9, no. 11 (2014). doi:10.1371/journal.pone.0112682.

202 Sigler ML, Stephens TJ. Assessment of the safety and efficacy of topical copper chlorophyllin in women with photodamaged facial skin. *J Drugs Dermatol*. 2015 Apr;14(4):401-

203 Kaler SG1. Neurodevelopment and brain growth in classic Menkes disease is influenced by age and symptomatology at initiation of copper treatment. *J Trace Elem Med Biol*. 2014 Oct;28(4):427-30. doi: 10.1016/j.jtemb.2014.08.008. Epub 2014 Aug 28.

204 Dykes P1. Increase in skin surface elasticity in normal volunteer subjects following the use of copper oxide impregnated socks. *Skin Res Technol*. 2015 Aug;21(3):272-7. doi: 10.1111/srt.12187. Epub 2014 Aug 16.

205 Dykes P1. Increase in skin surface elasticity in normal volunteer subjects following the use of copper oxide impregnated socks. *Skin Res Technol*. 2015 Aug;21(3):272-7. doi: 10.1111/srt.12187. Epub 2014 Aug 16.

206 Ala S1, Shokrzadeh M, Pur Shoja AM, Saeedi Saravi SS. Zinc and copper plasma concentrations in rheumatoid arthritis patients from a selected population in Iran. *Pak J Biol Sci*. 2009 Jul 15;12(14):1041-4.

207 Fatemi Naieni F1, Ebrahimi B, Vakilian HR, Shahmoradi Z. Serum iron, zinc, and copper concentration in premature graying of hair. *Biol Trace Elem Res*. 2012 Apr;146(1):30-4. doi: 10.1007/s12011-011-9223-6. Epub 2011 Oct 7.

208 Brewer GJ1. The risks of copper toxicity contributing to cognitive decline in the aging population and to Alzheimer's disease. *J Am Coll Nutr*. 2009 Jun;28(3):238-42.

[209] Wazir SM, Ghobrial I. Copper deficiency, a new triad: anemia, leucopenia, and myelonephropathy. J Community Hosp Intern Med Perspect. 2017 Sep 19;7(4):265-268. Doi: 10.1080/20009666.2017.1351289. eCollection 2017 Oct.

[210] Ambooken Betsy, MP Binitha, and S Sarita. Zinc Deficiency Associated with Hypothyroidism: An Overlooked Cause of Severe Alopecia

[211] DiSilvestro RA1, Joseph EL, Zhang W, Raimo AE, Kim YM. A randomized trial of copper supplementation effects on blood copper enzyme activities and parameters related to cardiovascular health. *Metabolism.* 2012 Sep;61(9):1242-6. doi: 10.1016/j.metabol.2012.02.002. Epub 2012 Mar 22.

[212] Shahrami, Ali, Farhad Assarzadegan, Hamid Reza Hatamabadi, Morteza Asgarzadeh, Baharak Sarehbandi, and Setareh Asgarzadeh. "Comparison of Therapeutic Effects of Magnesium Sulfate vs. Dexamethasone/Metoclopramide on Alleviating Acute Migraine Headache." *The Journal of Emergency Medicine* 48, no. 1 (2015): 69-76. doi:10.1016/j.jemermed.2014.06.055.

[213] Torres, Silvio. "Effectiveness of Magnesium Sulfate as Initial Treatment of Acute Severe Asthma in Children. A Randomized, Controlled Trial." *Arch Argent Pediat Archivos Argentinos De Pediatria* 110, no. 4 (2012): 291-97. doi:10.5546/aap.2012.eng.291.

[214] Ahsan, B. et al. "The Effects of Magnesium Sulphate on Succinylcholine-induced Fasciculation during Induction of General Anaesthesia." *J Pak Med Assoc.* 64, no. 10 (October 2014): 1151-153.

[215] Veronese, N., L. Berton, S. Carraro, F. Bolzetta, M. De Rui, E. Perissinotto, E. D. Toffanello, E. Bano, S. Pizzato, F. Miotto, A. Coin, E. Manzato, and G. Sergi. "Effect of Oral Magnesium Supplementation on Physical Performance in Healthy Elderly Women Involved in a Weekly Exercise Program: A Randomized Controlled Trial." *American Journal of Clinical Nutrition* 100, no. 3 (2014): 974-81. doi:10.3945/ajcn.113.080168.

[216] Setaro, Luciana, Paulo Roberto Santos-Silva, Eduardo Yoshio Nakano, Cristiane Hermes Sales, Newton Nunes, Júlia Maria Greve, and Célia Colli. "Magnesium Status and the Physical Performance of Volleyball Players:

Effects of Magnesium Supplementation." *Journal of Sports Sciences* 32, no. 5 (2013): 438-45. doi:10.1080/02640414.2013.828847.

[217] Supakatisant, Chayanis, and Vorapong Phupong. "Oral Magnesium for Relief in Pregnancy-induced Leg Cramps: A Randomised Controlled Trial." *Matern Child Nutr Maternal & Child Nutrition* 11, no. 2 (2012): 139-45. doi:10.1111/j.1740-8709.2012.00440.x.

[218] Aissaoui, Younes, Youssef Qamous, Issam Serghini, Mohammed Zoubir, Jaafar Lalaoui Salim, and Mohammed Boughalem. "Magnesium Sulphate." *European Journal of Anaesthesiology* 29, no. 8 (2012): 391-97. doi:10.1097/eja.0b013e328355cf35.

[219] Gontijo-Amaral, C., E. V. Guimaraes, and P. Camargos. "Oral Magnesium Supplementation in Children with Cystic Fibrosis Improves Clinical and Functional Variables: A Double-blind, Randomized, Placebo-controlled Crossover Trial." *American Journal of Clinical Nutrition* 96, no. 1 (2012): 50-56. doi:10.3945/ajcn.112.034207.

[220] Lee, Ae Ryoung, Hye-Won Yi, In Sun Chung, Justin Sangwook Ko, Hyun Joo Ahn, Mi Sook Gwak, Duck Hwan Choi, and Soo Joo Choi. "Magnesium Added to Bupivacaine Prolongs the Duration of Analgesia after Interscalene Nerve Block." *Can J Anesth/J Can Anesth Canadian Journal of Anesthesia/Journal Canadien D'anesthésie* 59, no. 1 (2011): 21-27. doi:10.1007/s12630-011-9604-5.

[221] Engen, Deborah J., Samantha J. Mcallister, Mary O. Whipple, Stephen S. Cha, Liza J. Dion, Ann Vincent, Brent A. Bauer, and Dietlind L. Wahner-Roedler. "Effects of Transdermal Magnesium Chloride on Quality of Life for Patients with Fibromyalgia: A Feasibility Study." *Journal of Integrative Medicine* 13, no. 5 (2015): 306-13. doi:10.1016/s2095-4964(15)60195-9.

[222] Guerrero-Romero, F., L.e. Simental-Mendía, G. Hernández-Ronquillo, and M. Rodriguez-Morán. "Oral Magnesium Supplementation Improves Glycaemic Status in Subjects with Prediabetes and Hypomagnesaemia: A Double-blind Placebo-controlled Randomized Trial." *Diabetes & Metabolism* 41, no. 3 (2015): 202-07. doi:10.1016/j.diabet.2015.03.010.

[223] Rabinovitz H1, Friedensohn A, Leibovitz A, Gabay G, Rocas C, Habot B. Effect of chromium supplementation on blood glucose and lipid levels in type 2 diabetes mellitus elderly patients. *Int J Vitam Nutr Res.* 2004 May;74(3):178-82.

[224] Stephen D. Anton, Ph.D.,1,,2 Christopher D. Morrison, Ph.D.,1 William T. Cefalu, M.D.,1 Corby K. Martin, Ph.D.,1Sandra Coulon, B.A.,1 Paula

Geiselman, Ph.D.,1,,3 Hongmei Han, M.S.,1 Christy L. White, D.V.M.,1 and Donald A. Williamson, Ph.D.1. Effects of Chromium Picolinate on Food Intake and Satiety

[225] Whitney Sealls,1 Brent A. Penque,1 and Jeffrey S. Elmendorf1,2. Evidence That Chromium Modulates Cellular Cholesterol Homeostasis and ABCA1 Functionality Impaired By Hyperinsulinemia

[226] Hummel M1, Standl E, Schnell O. Chromium in metabolic and cardiovascular disease. *Horm Metab Res.* 2007 Oct;39(10):743-51.

[227] Wallach S. Clinical and biochemical aspects of chromium deficiency. *J Am Coll Nutr.* 1985;4(1):107-20.

[228] McCarty MF1. Longevity effect of chromium picolinate--'rejuvenation' of hypothalamic function. *Med Hypotheses.* 1994 Oct;43(4):253-65.

[229] Yinan Hua, Suzanne Clark, Jun Ren, and Nair Sreejayan. Molecular Mechanisms of Chromium in Alleviating Insulin Resistance

[230] Head KA1. Peripheral neuropathy: pathogenic mechanisms and alternative therapies. *Altern Med Rev.* 2006 Dec;11(4):294-329.

[231] Lima KV1, Lima RP, Gonçalves MC, Faintuch J, Morais LC, Asciutti LS, Costa MJ. High frequency of serum chromium deficiency and association of chromium with triglyceride and cholesterol concentrations in patients awaiting bariatric surgery. *Obes Surg.* 2014 May;24(5):771-6. doi: 10.1007/s11695-013-1132-7.

[232] Pérez-Martínez P, Mikhailidis DP, et al. Lifestyle recommendations for the prevention and management of metabolic syndrome: an international panel recommendation. Nutr Rev. 2017 May 1;75(5):307-326. doi: 10.1093/nutrit/nux014.

[233] Hildebrandt W1, Sauer R2, Bonaterra G3, Dugi KA4, Edler L5, Kinscherf R3. Oral N-acetylcysteine reduces plasma homocysteine concentrations regardless of lipid or smoking status. *Am J Clin Nutr.* 2015 Nov;102(5):1014-24. doi: 10.3945/ajcn.114.101964. Epub 2015 Oct 7.

[234] Karelis AD1, Messier V, Suppère C, Briand P, Rabasa-Lhoret R. Effect of cysteine-rich whey protein (immunocal®) supplementation in combination with resistance training on muscle strength and lean body mass in non-frail elderly subjects: a randomized, double-blind controlled study. *J Nutr Health Aging.* 2015 May;19(5):531-6. doi: 10.1007/s12603-015-0442-y.

[235] Larsson SC1, Håkansson N2, Wolk A2. Dietary cysteine and other amino acids and stroke incidence in women.
*Stroke.* 2015 Apr;46(4):922-6. doi: 10.1161/STROKEAHA.114.008022. Epub 2015 Feb 10.

[236] Nikoo M1, Radnia H, Farokhnia M, Mohammadi MR, Akhondzadeh S. N-acetylcysteine as an adjunctive therapy to risperidone for treatment of irritability in autism: a randomized, double-blind, placebo-controlled clinical trial of efficacy and safety. *Clin Neuropharmacol.* 2015 Jan-Feb;38(1):11-7. doi: 10.1097/WNF.0000000000000063.

[237] Kuyumcu A, Akyol A, Buyuktuncer Z, Ozmen MM, Besler HT1. Improved oxidative status in major abdominal surgery patients after N-acetyl cystein supplementation. *Nutr J.* 2015 Jan 6;14:4. doi: 10.1186/1475-2891-14-4.

[238] Conrad C1, Lymp J2, Thompson V2, Dunn C1, Davies Z1, Chatfield B3, Nichols D4, Clancy J5, Vender R6, Egan ME7, Quittell L8, Michelson P9, Antony V10,Spahr J11, Rubenstein RC12, Moss RB1, Herzenberg LA13, Goss CH2, Tirouvanziam R14. Long-term treatment with oral N-acetylcysteine: affects lung function but not sputum inflammation in cystic fibrosis subjects. A phase II randomized placebo-controlled trial. *J Cyst Fibros.* 2015 Mar;14(2):219-27. doi: 10.1016/j.jcf.2014.08.008. Epub 2014 Sep 13.

[239] Vidart J1, Wajner SM, Leite RS, Manica A, Schaan BD, Larsen PR, Maia AL. N-acetylcysteine administration prevents nonthyroidal illness syndrome in patients with acute myocardial infarction: a randomized clinical trial. *J Clin Endocrinol Metab.* 2014 Dec;99(12):4537-45. doi: 10.1210/jc.2014-2192.

[240] Georgina Oliver,1 Olivia Dean,1,2,3 David Camfield,4,5,6 Scott Blair-West,1 Chee Ng,1 Michael Berk,1,2,3,4 and Jerome Sarris1,4. N-Acetyl Cysteine in the Treatment of Obsessive Compulsive and Related Disorders: A Systematic Review

[241] Olivia Dean, BSc, PhD, Frank Giorlando, MBBS, BMedSc, and Michael Berk, MBBCh, MMed(Psych), PhD N-acetylcysteine in psychiatry: current therapeutic evidence and potential mechanisms of action

[242] Rushworth GF1, Megson IL2. Existing and potential therapeutic uses for N-acetylcysteine: the need for conversion to intracellular glutathione for antioxidant benefits. *Pharmacol Ther.* 2014 Feb;141(2):150-9. doi: 10.1016/j.pharmthera.2013.09.006. Epub 2013 Sep 28.

243 Salehpour S1, Sene AA, Saharkhiz N, Sohrabi MR, Moghimian F. N-Acetylcysteine as an adjuvant to clomiphene citrate for successful induction of ovulation in infertile patients with polycystic ovary syndrome. *J Obstet Gynaecol Res.* 2012 Sep;38(9):1182-6. doi: 10.1111/j.1447-0756.2012.01844.x. Epub 2012 Apr 30.

244 Marazzi, Giuseppe, Francesco Pelliccia, Giuseppe Campolongo, Silvia Quattrino, Luca Cacciotti, Maurizio Volterrani, Carlo Gaudio, and Giuseppe Rosano. "Usefulness of Nutraceuticals (Armolipid Plus) Versus Ezetimibe and Combination in Statin-Intolerant Patients With Dyslipidemia With Coronary Heart Disease." *The American Journal of Cardiology* 116, no. 12 (2015): 1798-801. doi:10.1016/j.amjcard.2015.09.023.

245 Šabovič, Mišo. "Coenzyme Q10 Supplementation Decreases Statin-Related Mild-to-Moderate Muscle Symptoms: A Randomized Clinical Study." *Med Sci Monit Medical Science Monitor* 20 (2014): 2183-2188. doi:10.12659/msm.890777.

246 Mortensen, Svend A., Franklin Rosenfeldt, Adarsh Kumar, Peter Dolliner, Krzysztof J. Filipiak, Daniel Pella, Urban Alehagen, Günter Steurer, and Gian P. Littarru. "The Effect of Coenzyme Q10 on Morbidity and Mortality in Chronic Heart Failure." *JACC: Heart Failure* 2, no. 6 (2014): 641-49. doi:10.1016/j.jchf.2014.06.008.

247 Langsjoen, Peter H., and Alena M. Langsjoen. "Supplemental Ubiquinol in Patients with Advanced Congestive Heart Failure." *BioFactors* 32, no. 1-4 (2008): 119-28. doi:10.1002/biof.5520320114.

248 Burke, Briant E., Roger Neuenschwander, and Richard D. Olson. "Randomized, Double-Blind, Placebo- Controlled Trial of Coenzyme Q10 in Isolated Systolic Hypertension." *Southern Medical Journal* 94, no. 11 (2001): 1112-1117. doi:10.1097/00007611-200111000-00015.

249 Gvozdjáková, Anna, Jarmila Kucharská, Daniela Ostatníková, Katarína Babinská, Dalibor Nakládal, and Fred L. Crane. "Ubiquinol Improves Symptoms in Children with Autism." *Oxidative Medicine and Cellular Longevity* 2014 (2014): 1-6. doi:10.1155/2014/798957.

250 Refaeey, Abdelaziz El, Amal Selem, and Ahmed Badawy. "Combined Coenzyme Q10 and Clomiphene Citrate for Ovulation Induction in Clomiphene-citrate-resistant Polycystic Ovary Syndrome." *Reproductive BioMedicine Online* 29, no. 1 (2014): 119-24. doi:10.1016/j.rbmo.2014.03.011.

251 Gaul, Charly, Hans-Christoph Diener, and Ulrich Danesch. "Improvement of Migraine Symptoms with a Proprietary Supplement Containing Riboflavin,

Magnesium and Q10: A Randomized, Placebo-controlled, Double-blind, Multicenter Trial." *J Headache Pain The Journal of Headache and Pain* 16, no. 1 (2015). doi:10.1186/s10194-015-0516-6.

252 Hertz, N., and R. Lister. "Improved Survival in Patients with End-Stage Cancer Treated with Coenzyme Q10 and Other Antioxidants: A Pilot Study." *Journal of International Medical Research* 37, no. 6 (2009): 1961-971. doi:10.1177/147323000903700634.

253 Lockwood, K., S. Moesgaard, and K. Folkers. "Partial and Complete Regression of Breast Cancer in Patients in Relation to Dosage of Coenzyme Q10." *Biochemical and Biophysical Research Communications* 199, no. 3 (1994): 1504-508. doi:10.1006/bbrc.1994.1401.

254 Asemi Z1, Jamilian M2, Mesdaghinia E3, Esmaillzadeh A4. Effects of selenium supplementation on glucose homeostasis, inflammation, and oxidative stress in gestational diabetes: Randomized, double-blind, placebo-controlled trial. *Nutrition.* 2015 Oct;31(10):1235-42. doi: 10.1016/j.nut.2015.04.014. Epub 2015 May 14.

255 Vieira ML1, Fonseca FL, Costa LG, Beltrame RL, Chaves CM, Cartum J, Alves SI, Azzalis LA, Junqueira VB, Pereria EC, Rocha KC. Supplementation with selenium can influence nausea, fatigue, physical, renal, and liver function of children and adolescents with cancer. *J Med Food.* 2015 Jan;18(1):109-17. doi: 10.1089/jmf.2014.0030.

256 Alvarenga Americano do Brasil PE1, Pereira de Souza A, Hasslocher-Moreno AM, Xavier SS, Lambert Passos SR, de Fátima Ramos Moreira M, Santini de Oliveira M, Sperandio da Silva GM, Magalhães Saraiva R, Santos de Aguiar Cardoso C, de Sousa AS, Mediano MF, Bonecini de Almeida Mda G, da Cruz Moreira O, Britto C, de Araújo-Jorge TC. Selenium Treatment and Chagasic Cardiopathy (STCC): study protocol for a double-blind randomized controlled trial. *Trials.* 2014 Oct 6;15:388. doi: 10.1186/1745-6215-15-388.

257 O'Dell JR1, Lemley-Gillespie S, Palmer WR, Weaver AL, Moore GF, Klassen LW. Serum selenium concentrations in rheumatoid arthritis. *Ann Rheum Dis.* 1991 Jun;50(6):376-8.

258 Yu N1, Han F1, Lin X1, Tang C1, Ye J1, Cai X2. The Association Between Serum Selenium Levels with Rheumatoid Arthritis. *Biol Trace Elem Res.* 2016 Jul;172(1):46-52. Epub 2015 Nov 18.

[259] Rayman MP1. Selenium in cancer prevention: a review of the evidence and mechanism of action. *Proc Nutr Soc.* 2005 Nov;64(4):527-42.

[260] Yu-Chi Chen,1 K. Sandeep Prabhu,2,3,4 and Andrea M. Mastro. Is Selenium a Potential Treatment for Cancer Metastasis?

[261] Drutel A1, Archambeaud F, Caron P. Selenium and the thyroid gland: more good news for clinicians. *Clin Endocrinol (Oxf).* 2013 Feb;78(2):155-64. doi: 10.1111/cen.12066.

[262] Ashley N. Ogawa-Wong,* Marla J. Berry, and Lucia A. Seale Selenium and Metabolic Disorders: An Emphasis on Type 2 Diabetes Risk

[263] Mohammad K Moslemi1,2 and Samaneh Tavanbakhsh. Selenium–vitamin E supplementation in infertile men: effects on semen parameters and pregnancy rate

[264] Pillai R1, Uyehara-Lock JH, Bellinger FP. Selenium and selenoprotein function in brain disorders. *IUBMB Life.* 2014 Apr;66(4):229-39. doi: 10.1002/iub.1262. Epub 2014 Mar 25.

[265] Takemoto D1, Yasutake Y, Tomimori N, Ono Y, Shibata H, Hayashi J. Sesame Lignans and Vitamin E Supplementation Improve Subjective Statuses and Anti-Oxidative Capacity in Healthy Humans With Feelings of Daily Fatigue. *Glob J Health Sci.* 2015 Mar 25;7(6):1-10. doi: 10.5539/gjhs.v7n6p1.

[266] Yousefichaijan P, Kahbazi M, Rasti S, Rafeie M, Sharafkhah M1. Vitamin E as adjuvant treatment for urinary tract infection in girls with acute pyelonephritis. *Iran J Kidney Dis.* 2015 Mar;9(2):97-104.

[267] Shamim AA1, Schulze K1, Merrill RD1, Kabir A1, Christian P1, Shaikh S1, Wu L1, Ali H1, Labrique AB1, Mehra S1, Klemm RD1, Rashid M1, Sungpuag P1,Udomkesmalee E1, West KP Jr1. First-trimester plasma tocopherols are associated with risk of miscarriage in rural Bangladesh. *Am J Clin Nutr.* 2015 Feb;101(2):294-301. doi: 10.3945/ajcn.114.094920. Epub 2014 Nov 26.

[268] Farris P, Yatskayer M, Chen N, Krol Y, Oresajo C. Evaluation of efficacy and tolerance of a nighttime topical antioxidant containing resveratrol, baicalin, andvitamin e for treatment of mild to moderately photodamaged skin. *J Drugs Dermatol.* 2014 Dec;13(12):1467-72.

[269] Remington R1, Bechtel C2, Larsen D3, Samar A4, Doshanjh L5, Fishman P6, Luo Y6, Smyers K1, Page R2, Morrell C5, Shea TB1. A Phase II Randomized Clinical Trial of a Nutritional Formulation for Cognition and

Mood in Alzheimer's Disease. *J Alzheimers Dis.* 2015;45(2):395-405. doi: 10.3233/JAD-142499.

[270] Bunchorntavakul C, Wootthananont T, Atsawarungruangkit A. Effects of vitamin E on chronic hepatitis C genotype 3: a randomized, double-blind, placebo-controlled study. *J Med Assoc Thai.* 2014 Nov;97 Suppl 11:S31-40.

[271] Hajar Dadkhah,1 Elham Ebrahimi,2 and Nahid Fathizadeh1. Evaluating the effects of vitamin D and vitamin E supplement on premenstrual syndrome: A randomized, double-blind, controlled trial

[272] Saliha Rizvi, Syed T. Raza,* Faizal Ahmed, Absar Ahmad, Shania Abbas, and Farzana Mahdi. The Role of Vitamin E in Human Health and Some Diseases

[273] Wada S1. Cancer preventive effects of vitamin E. *Curr Pharm Biotechnol.* 2012 Jan;13(1):156-64.

[274] Mocchegiani E1, Costarelli L2, Giacconi R2, Malavolta M2, Basso A2, Piacenza F2, Ostan R3, Cevenini E3, Gonos ES4, Franceschi C3, Monti D5. Vitamin E-gene interactions in aging and inflammatory age-related diseases: implications for treatment. A systematic review. *Ageing Res Rev.* 2014 Mar;14:81-101. doi: 10.1016/j.arr.2014.01.001. Epub 2014 Jan 11.

[275] Scaramuzza A1, Giani E2, Redaelli F2, Ungheri S2, Macedoni M2, Giudici V2, Bosetti A1, Ferrari M1, Zuccotti GV2. Alpha-Lipoic Acid and Antioxidant Diet Help to Improve Endothelial Dysfunction in Adolescents with Type 1 Diabetes: A Pilot Trial. *J Diabetes Res.* 2015;2015:474561. doi: 10.1155/2015/474561. Epub 2015 Jun 16.

[276] Haghighian HK1, Haidari F2, Mohammadi-Asl J3, Dadfar M4. Randomized, triple-blind, placebo-controlled clinical trial examining the effects of alpha-lipoic acid supplement on the spermatogram and seminal oxidative stress in infertile men. *Fertil Steril.* 2015 Aug;104(2):318-24. doi: 10.1016/j.fertnstert.2015.05.014. Epub 2015 Jun 11.

[277] Gerritje S. Mijnhout, 1 ,* Boudewijn J. Kollen, 2 Alaa Alkhalaf, 1 ,3 ,4 Nanno Kleefstra, 3 ,4 ,5 and Henk J. G. Bilo. Alpha Lipoic Acid for Symptomatic Peripheral Neuropathy in Patients with Diabetes: A Meta-Analysis of Randomized Controlled Trials

[278] Ansar H1, Mazloom Z, Kazemi F, Hejazi N. Effect of alpha-lipoic acid on blood glucose, insulin resistance and glutathione peroxidase of type 2 diabetic patients. *Saudi Med J.* 2011 Jun;32(6):584-8.

[279] Koriyama Y1, Nakayama Y, Matsugo S, Kato S. Protective effect of lipoic acid against oxidative stress is mediated by Keap1/Nrf2-dependent heme oxygenase-1 induction in the RGC-5 cellline. *Brain Res.* 2013 Mar 7;1499:145-57. doi: 10.1016/j.brainres.2012.12.041. Epub 2013 Jan 4.

[280] Midaoui AE1, Elimadi A, Wu L, Haddad PS, de Champlain J. Lipoic acid prevents hypertension, hyperglycemia, and the increase in heart mitochondrial superoxide production. *Am J Hypertens.* 2003 Mar;16(3):173-9.

[281] Jariwalla RJ1, Lalezari J, Cenko D, Mansour SE, Kumar A, Gangapurkar B, Nakamura D. Restoration of blood total glutathione status and lymphocyte function following alpha-lipoic acidsupplementation in patients with HIV infection. *J Altern Complement Med.* 2008 Mar;14(2):139-46. doi: 10.1089/acm.2006.6397.

[282] Puizina-Ivić N1, Mirić L, Carija A, Karlica D, Marasović D. Modern approach to topical treatment of aging skin. *Coll Antropol.* 2010 Sep;34(3):1145-53.

[283] Durand M1, Mach N. [Alpha lipoic acid and its antioxidant against cancer and diseases of central sensitization].
[Article in Spanish] *Nutr Hosp.* 2013 Jul Aug;28(4).1031-8. doi: 10.3305/nh.2013.28.4.6589.

[284] Durand M1, Mach N. [Alpha lipoic acid and its antioxidant against cancer and diseases of central sensitization].
[Article in Spanish] *Nutr Hosp.* 2013 Jul-Aug;28(4):1031-8. doi: 10.3305/nh.2013.28.4.6589.

[285] Oliveira, Ivaldo Jesus Lima De, Victor Vasconcelos De Souza, Vitor Motta, and Sergio Leme Da-Silva. "Effects of Oral Vitamin C Supplementation on Anxiety in Students: A Double-Blind, Randomized, Placebo-Controlled Trial." *Pakistan J. of Biological Sciences Pakistan Journal of Biological Sciences* 18, no. 1 (2015): 11-18. doi:10.3923/pjbs.2015.11.18.

[286] Sasazuki, S., S. Sasaki, Y. Tsubono, S. Okubo, M. Hayashi, and S. Tsugane. "Effect of Vitamin C on Common Cold: Randomized Controlled Trial." *European Journal of Clinical Nutrition Eur J Clin Nutr* 60, no. 1 (2005): 9-17. doi:10.1038/sj.ejcn.1602261.

[287] Besse, Jean-Luc, Sylvain Gadeyne, Sophie Galand-Desmé, Jean-Luc Lerat, and Bernard Moyen. "Effect of Vitamin C on Prevention of Complex

Regional Pain Syndrome Type I in Foot and Ankle Surgery." *Foot and Ankle Surgery* 15, no. 4 (2009): 179-82. doi:10.1016/j.fas.2009.02.002.

288 Barbosa, Eliana, Joel Faintuch, Emilia Addison Machado Moreira, Viviane Rodrigues Gonçalves Da Silva, Maurício José Lopes Pereima, Regina Lúcia Martins Fagundes, and Danilo Wilhelm Filho. "Supplementation of Vitamin E, Vitamin C, and Zinc Attenuates Oxidative Stress in Burned Children: A Randomized, Double-Blind, Placebo-Controlled Pilot Study." *Journal of Burn Care & Research* 30, no. 5 (2009): 859-66. doi:10.1097/bcr.0b013e3181b487a8.

289 Ohshima, Hiroshi, Koji Mizukoshi, Midori Oyobikawa, Katsuo Matsumoto, Hirotsugu Takiwaki, Hiromi Kanto, and Masatoshi Itoh. "Effects of Vitamin C on Dark Circles of the Lower Eyelids: Quantitative Evaluation Using Image Analysis and Echogram." *Skin Research and Technology* 15, no. 2 (2009): 214-17. doi:10.1111/j.1600-0846.2009.00356.x.

290 Haftek, Marek, Sophie Mac-Mary, Marie-Aude Le Bitoux, Pierre Creidi, Sophie Seité, André Rougier, and Philippe Humbert. "Clinical, Biometric and Structural Evaluation of the Long-term Effects of a Topical Treatment with Ascorbic Acid and Madecassoside in Photoaged Human Skin." *Experimental Dermatology* 17, no. 11 (2008): 946-52. doi:10.1111/j.1600-0625.2008.00732.x.

291 Hoffer, L. John, Line Robitaille, Robert Zakarian, David Melnychuk, Petr Kavan, Jason Agulnik, Victor Cohen, David Small, and Wilson H. Miller. "High-Dose Intravenous Vitamin C Combined with Cytotoxic Chemotherapy in Patients with Advanced Cancer: A Phase I-II Clinical Trial." *PLOS ONE PLoS ONE* 10, no. 4 (2015). doi:10.1371/journal.pone.0120228.

292 Garaiova, I., J. Muchová, Z. Nagyová, D. Wang, J. V. Li, Z. Országhová, D. R. Michael, S. F. Plummer, and Z. Ďuračková. "Probiotics and Vitamin C for the Prevention of Respiratory Tract Infections in Children Attending Preschool: A Randomised Controlled Pilot Study." *European Journal of Clinical Nutrition Eur J Clin Nutr* 69, no. 3 (2014): 373-79. doi:10.1038/ejcn.2014.174.

293 Kim, M., H. Yang, H. Kim, H. Jung, and H. Jung. "Novel Cosmetic Patches for Wrinkle Improvement: Retinyl Retinoate- and Ascorbic Acid-loaded Dissolving Microneedles." *International Journal of Cosmetic Science Int J Cosmet Sci* 36, no. 3 (2014): 207-12. doi:10.1111/ics.12115.

[294] Casanueva, E. et al. "Vitamin C Supplementation to Prevent Premature Rupture of the Chorioamniotic Membranes: A Randomized Trial." *Am J Clin Nutr.* 81, no. 4 (April 2005): 859-63.

[295] Yuasa M, Matsui T, et al. Consumption of a low-carbohydrate and high-fat diet (the ketogenic diet) exaggerates biotin deficiency in mice. Nutrition. 2013 Oct;29(10):1266-70. doi: 10.1016/j.nut.2013.04.011.

[296] Schugar RC, Huang X, Moll AR, Brunt EM, Crawford PA. Role of choline deficiency in the Fatty liver phenotype of mice fed a low protein, very low carbohydrate ketogenic diet. PLoS One. 2013 Aug 29;8(8):e74806. doi: 10.1371/journal.pone.0074806. eCollection 2013.

[297] Hua Y, Clark S, Ren J, Sreejayan N. Molecular mechanisms of chromium in alleviating insulin resistance. J Nutr Biochem. 2012 Apr;23(4):313-9. doi: 10.1016/j.jnutbio.2011.11.001.

[298] Beigi Harchegani A, Dahan H, et al. Effects of zinc deficiency on impaired spermatogenesis and male infertility: the role of oxidative stress, inflammation and apoptosis. Hum Fertil (Camb). 2018 Aug 21:1-12. doi: 10.1080/14647273.2018.1494390.

[299] Bager P. Fatigue and acute/chronic anaemia. Dan Med J. 2014 Apr;61(4):B4824.

[300] Yao Y, Fu S, et al. The prevalence of depressive symptoms in Chinese longevous persons and its correlation with vitamin D status. BMC Geriatr. 2018 Aug 29;18(1):198. doi: 10.1186/s12877-018-0886-0.

[301] Coppen A, Bolander-Gouaille C. Treatment of depression: time to consider folic acid and vitamin B12. J Psychopharmacol. 2005 Jan;19(1):59-65.

[302] Özkaya F, Demirel A. Vitamin D deficiency in infertile patients. Arch Esp Urol. 2018 Dec;71(10):850-855.

[303] Yang GT, Zhao HY, Kong Y, Sun NN, Dong AQ. Correlation between serum vitamin B12 level and peripheral neuropathy in atrophic gastritis. World J Gastroenterol. 2018 Mar 28;24(12):1343-1352. doi: 10.3748/wjg.v24.i12.1343.

[304] Almohanna HM, Ahmed AA, Tsatalis JP, Tosti A. The Role of Vitamins and Minerals in Hair Loss: A Review. Dermatol Ther (Heidelb). 2018 Dec 13. doi: 10.1007/s13555-018-0278-6. [Epub ahead of print]

[305] Wen L, Chen J, Duan L, Li S. Vitamin K-dependent proteins involved in bone and cardiovascular health (Review). Mol Med Rep. 2018 Jul;18(1):3-15. doi: 10.3892/mmr.2018.8940. Epub 2018 Apr 27.